PRACTICAL

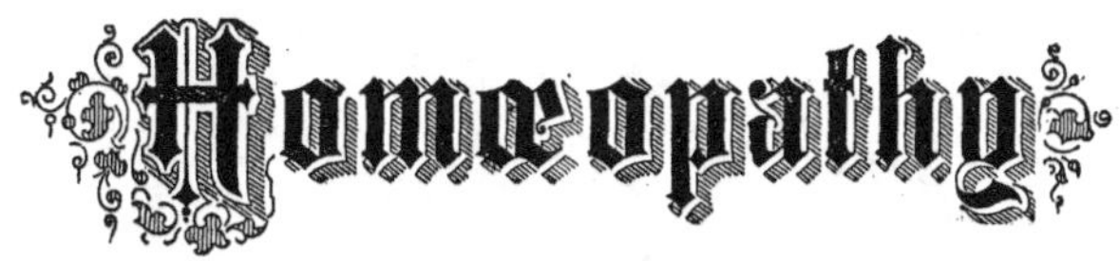

FOR THE PEOPLE:

ADAPTED TO THE COMPREHENSION OF THE NON-PROFESSIONAL, AND FOR REFERENCE BY THE YOUNG PRACTITIONER, INCLUDING A NUMBER OF MOST

VALUABLE NEW REMEDIES.

THIRTEENTH EDITION.

BY J. S. DOUGLAS, A. M., M. D., PH. D.

Late Professor of Mat. Med., Special Pathology and Diagnosis, in the Western Hom. Med. College, Cleveland, O.; Fellow and Corresponding Member of the Penn. Hom. Medical College at Philadelphia.

AUTHOR OF

"Treatment of Intermittent Fever," "Homœopathy, its Principles and Practice Explained and Illustrated," "Modern Spiritualism, its Scientific and Moral Aspects," Etc., Etc.

MILWAUKEE, WIS.:
DOUGLAS & SHERMAN.
CHICAGO: HALSEY BROS.
1875.

Godfrey & Crandall, Printers, Milwaukee.

PREFACE.

In furnishing the public with Homœopathic remedies, with directions for their use, it is proper to state the motives for so doing. These are:

FIRST.—A knowledge of the vast superiority of Homœopathic treatment over the old system.

SECOND.—A large portion of the population, of the West especially, are not within reach of a Homœopathic physician, and, if they employ the remedies, are obliged to depend upon such knowledge of them as they can acquire from books designed for domestic use.

THIRD.—The reputation of Homœopathic remedies has become so general, and the demand for them so great, that the country is becoming flooded with Homœopathic quackery, under the name of "Specific Homœopathic Remedies," no one knowing what they are but him who prepares them. When a bottle or box is exhausted, the owner has no resource but to send to the getter-up of these nostrums, or some of his agents, to get it replenished. The unfortunate example of this mode of quackery has been set by a medical man at the East, who has thereby forfeited his standing in the profession, and been, very properly, expelled from the American Institute. His example is being followed by others, who have a higher regard for their own pockets than for their professional reputation or the interests of the public.

All reasoning persons will prefer to know what the medicines are which they use, and when one is exhausted, to be able to replenish it at any place where Homœopathic medicines are kept, and at the same time enjoy the practical benefits of knowing what the remedies are which effect cures of different diseases.

Besides these considerations, any reasoning person, by a moment's reflection, will be convinced how totally inadequate these "Specifics" are to cure all the diseases for which they are advertised, and how unsafe it must be to trust them. We have no hesitation in saying to the public that it is totally unsafe to trust to these "Specific Remedies" for the treatment of the various diseases for which they are prescribed, as much so as to trust the thousand other mixtures advertised to cure everything.

I do not aim to make accomplished physicians of the public, nor expect that *every* case of disease can be safely treated domestically. But I do know, from numerous examples of domestic practice, that a long catalogue of acute and serious diseases, as well as lighter disorders, will be treated much more safely and successfully by families, by following the directions here given, than they are treated by the best drugging physicians.

Nor is it my design to treat of every disease to which humanity is subject, nor to prescribe every remedy of the Materia Medica. But I shall give brief and unmistakable directions for *curing* the great mass of diseases of the country, constituting nine-tenths of all the cases for which the physician is usually consulted, with remedies enough to meet those cases, *among which are a considerable number of most valuable and even indispensable remedies, which have been recently introduced.*

It is greatly to be regretted that so many Allopathic physicians are dabbling with Homœopathic remedies, and pretending that they can practice Homœopathy where it is appropriate, as well as we, without any of the study or knowledge necessary to use them with any success or credit to the system. When by their bungling misapplication of these beautiful remedies, they fail of success, or, by giving them in Allopathic doses, do serious mischief, they pronounce Homœopathy, not adapted to such cases. As well might a bungler, after spoiling a board and mangling his hand, by attempting to use a saw, pronounce a saw not adapted for use.

In short, my one great object in this issue of medicines, with appropriate directions, is to make known and extend the blessings of Homœopathic remedies properly applied, by bringing the community to a practical acquaintance with them, and inducing them to witness their beneficent effects under their own administration and experience. I hope that very many who have never used Homœopathic remedies will be induced to make the trial.

It will not be deemed egotistical by those who know him, or know of him, to say that this work is written by one who has devoted over forty years to the *study* as well as the *practice* of medicine, and who, in his intercourse with the best and most progressive physicians of the day, and in the performance of his duties as a teacher of medicine, the reading of the latest practical works, and the habitual proving of the new remedies on himself, and others, has anxiously labored to collect practical information, and apply it to the treatment of disease.

PREFACE TO 12TH EDITION.

This little book, in its first edition, was intended merely as a directory for the treatment of the most common diseases, to accompany family medicine chests, so much needed in the West, where Homœopathic physicians were not accessible. It was not offered or intended for sale. But dealers and physicians who happened to see a stray copy, applied for it, and urged its publication, somewhat enlarged, for the market. The author yielded to these solicitations, and the 12th edition of the unpretentious work is now demanded. By the advice of dealers and judicious medical friends, the present edition is considerably enlarged, embracing diseases not treated in former editions, and other additional matter. The author has always been partial to *small* plain works for domestic use. There are but few amateurs who want a large work. To the mass they are but puzzles and stumbling blocks. This little work is designed for the million, and is, therefore, written in such language as to be understood by them.

INTRODUCTION.

Most persons who have not given special attention to Homœopathy have very mistaken notions of it. It is very commonly thought to consist in giving very small doses. If an Allopathic physician gives very small doses, it is thought that he is almost Homœopathic. This is a great mistake. One may give just as small doses as we do, and yet make no approach to being Homœopathic. Homœopathy consists in treating disease according to a certain fixed law of cure. This law is expressed by the phrase, "LIKE CURES LIKE." The meaning of this phrase is, that a medicine in small doses will cure a disease, the like of which the same medicine will produce on a healthy person if given in large doses. The first inquiry which we make, when called to treat a disease is, "What medicine will produce a disease like it, in a healthy person, if given in large doses?" When we find such a remedy, we give it with entire confidence of success, if the disease is curable. The correctness of this law any one can prove on himself. For example, after one has seen fevers cured in a few hours by *Gelseminum*, in doses of half or quarter of a drop, let him test the correctness of the law, by taking, when he is well, five or ten drops of the same remedy. If he is at all sensitive, he will find, within five minutes, that his pulse has from ten to fifteen or twenty beats fewer in the minute, than it had before; and he will feel more or less chilly and dull. This will soon be followed by heat, quick pulse, flushed face, fullness and pain of the head, and perhaps pain of the back and limbs. In short he will feel that he has got a fever. Soon a prickling of the skin is felt, and a sweat breaks out, and after a few hours, he is well again. Now, it is just because Gelseminum *produces* a fever in LARGE doses, that it *cures* a similar fever in SMALL doses. The first dose I ever took of this remedy, when I was in perfect health, I *knew* that it would cure our prevalent fevers, as well as I know it now, after curing hundreds with it, because I knew that the law of "like cures like" was a true and reliable law. This is the law that guides us in all our treatment of disease. Every remedy prescribed in this book, for particular diseases, is prescribed, because it *produces* a similar disease. This is the secret of our great success, in the most formidable and dangerous diseases; a success that often astonishes those who do not understand the secret. Allopathic physicians have no such law to guide them. The only law that they have for treating disease is, the "cut and try" law, or the law of experiment, and all their experiments are made upon the sick, and at their expense. Our experiments are made before-hand on the healthy, and we enter at once on the *cure* of the sick, while they are *experimenting* upon them. Ours is a certain science—theirs is an uncertain art.

It will be readily seen that we cannot safely give large doses. If we did, we should produce the diseases we now cure. The accuracy of this law is proved to a demonstration, and every one may satisfy himself of it, a layman as well as a physician. And if this is a true law, then the practice of Homœopathy is a true practice, and all others are false. A most intelligent clergyman was investigating the truth of this law, and one day called and related the following case:

Said he, "In my younger days I was in the habit of drinking wine. I have a most vivid recollection of the bursting headache, the parched mouth, the burning thirst, the nausea, and the prostration the morning after a hard night's drinking. I awoke a few mornings since with all the feelings in a most distressing degree, though I had drank nothing. I related my feelings to my wife, saying that I felt exactly as if I had a night's debauch on wine. She laughingly replied that a Homœopathic dose of wine ought to cure me. I thought it a good chance to test the truth of the principle. I took two drops of wine in some water, and the effect was more remarkable than I ever witnessed from a dose of medicine. In five minutes my mouth was moist, my thirst abated, my headache vanishing, my strength returning, and in fifteen minutes I was perfectly well."

Here was a beautiful illustration of the law. A minute dose—two drops of wine—cured in a prompt and truly Homœopathic manner, a formidable train of symptoms, *like* those produced by large doses of the same article. This is equally true of all remedies. Tea produces, in those not accustomed to its use, anxiety, trembling, weakness, and palpitation of the heart; yet every lady knows that tea, in moderate quantity, is an excellent remedy for those very symptoms. Allopathic medical authorities furnish a thousand examples which proves this very law, though they do not understand it.

Tobacco, according to all Allopathic authorities, both produces and cures giddiness, nausea, trembling and weakness; *agaricus* produces and cures epilepsy; *belladonna* both produces and cures delirium and headache; *ipecac* and *antimony* produce and cure nausea and vomiting; *nitric acid*, *iodine* and *mercury* produce and cure salivation and ulceration of the mouth. We might fill a volume with similar examples. Large doses produce diseases—small ones cure them. It may seem strange to those who have never looked at the subject, that the same remedy should act in in such contrary directions, and produce and cure the same affections. It is, nevertheless, founded on nature and reason, which is more than can be said of most medical doctrines.

As I am desirous that every man and woman who reads this book, should know more of the philosophy of medicine than Allopathic physicians do, and to be able to meet the argument brought by them against Homœopathy, I propose to explain the philosophy of this Homœopathic law, so that all will understand it.

It is founded on the law of life—a vital principle. Let us question nature in this, as in all other things. My hands are cold, and I plunge them into cold water, or rub them in snow, and what is the result? In a few minutes they are glowing with warmth. This is not a freak of nature. Nature has no freaks. Her laws are uniform and universal, and this is an example of one of her laws. Take another example: My hands are hot, and I plunge them into hot water, and after a minute's exposure to the air, they become cool. Take other and varied examples: I burn my hand; it is hot, red, inflamed, and painful. On Allopathic principles, we should apply cold to remove this heat. And what would be the effect? Why, the heat and pain would be relieved for a short time, but the vital principle of reaction is aroused against it, and the hand soon becomes more hot, red, and painful than before. Hence, experience, without a knowledge of the law, has taught the profession that cold applications to a burn, though comfortable temporary palliatives, are very bad curatives. But adopt an opposite treatment, and apply a heating stimulant, as alcohol, or spirits of turpentine, or soft soap : the vital principle reacts against this, also, and in a short time, the heat, pain, and inflammation subside, a comfortable coolness follows, and the burn is soon cured.

A restless patient is put to sleep on opium, but on the following night he is more restless and sleepless than before. We might give a thousand examples of similar character.

This will enable us to understand two universal and practical laws, of the action of remedies, which the community should understand, if physicians do not. Such an understanding will do away with an immense amount of all-pervading and mischievous quackery.

First Law. Every medicine produces two directly opposite effects, in the order of time. The first, the primary and transient effect; the second, the secondary and more permanent one.

To illustrate this law by example: A patient takes a cathartic or a laxative. Its first, or primary effect, is to stimulate the intestines to unusual and unnatural activity; so much so, that he has, during its action, a medicinal diarrhœa. But this effect is transient, lasting only a few hours. Then comes the secondary effect, which is exactly the opposite, viz: unnatural inactivity and torpor, producing constipation.

Another illustration: Opium or morphine is

given to allay pain, and procure rest and sleep. This purpose is answered by its primary effect; but this soon ceases, and then comes the opposite, or secondary effect, that is, increased sensibility, restlessness and sleeplessness; and this is increased with every dose.

What is true of these two remedies, is true of all others. Yet this is the strange principle on which all Allopathic prescriptions are made, that is, to get the primary effects of medicines, which, if good, are at the best but very brief, and are soon followed by the opposite effect, which, of course, must be bad. Everybody is familiar with the fact, that multitudes of persons, after an Allopathic treatment, are left with lasting ruinous medicinal diseases, though the medicines may have done them temporary good.

If the public were thoroughly acquainted with this one law, they would never tolerate another dose of Allopathic medicine for themselves or for their families. If the physician should prescribe a laxative or cathartic, to remove constipation, the better informed patient would say to him something like this: "My dear sir, as I understand the laws of cure, your dose will give me very transient relief by its primary effect; but the secondary effect will be just the reverse, and will be lasting, so that I shall get only temporary relief, at the expense of a lasting aggravation of the very difficulty from which you propose to relieve me. I really cannot afford to pay such a price for so small a benefit." The same reasoning applies equally to every Allopathic prescription for every disease.

SECOND LAW. But there is another law, equally practical, and equally important, viz: That all medicines produce two exactly opposite effects, according to quantity; that is, small and large doses produce precisely opposite effects. So far is it from being true, that if a small dose will do a little good, a large one will do more, the truth is, that if a small dose does good, a large one will certainly do mischief, for the effects of the two are just the opposite of each other. For example: a small dose of *opium* produces wakefulness and exhilaration, while a large dose produces stupor and sleep. Small doses of *rhubarb*, *mercury*, and other cathartics, allay irritability of the bowels, and cure diarrhœa and dysentery, while large doses, everybody knows, produce precisely opposite effects. Very small doses of *ipecac.* or *tartar emetic*, allay irritation of the stomach, and stop vomiting and cholera morbus, while large doses produce only irritation and vomiting. The one is the disease-curing, the other disease-producing, effect.

Guided by this law, the physician will so administer his medicines as to secure the disease-curing effect, and avoid the disease-producing effect. Patients, well informed, will be wise enough to refuse a prescription made in violation of this law. But the Allopathic physician always aims to get the primary, or disease-producing effect. He knows nothing of treating disease by any other method. A wise patient will say to a physician who prescribes for him a large dose of medicine, (and *all* Allopathic doses are large, though they call them small): "Sir, I consulted you for the purpose of being cured, and you offer me a drug in a dose that will make me sick. The law of cure, as I understand it, makes it no part of the business of a physician to produce disease, but his exclusive business is to cure it. The time is past, when the appropriate inscription on a physician's sign was 'Disease Manufactory,' and the proper title of the profession, 'The *destructive* art of healing.' I must insist on your treating me in harmony with the now well-known laws of cure, or I must take the treatment into my own hands, or consult some one better informed."

We can now better understand the reason of the law, "LIKE CURES LIKE." We see a patient laboring under symptoms exactly like those produced by large doses of *Belladonna.* This, then, must be the appropriate remedy, because, in small doses, it produces symptoms exactly the opposite of those produced by large doses, and the opposite of those under which the patient labors, and, of course, establishes an opposite effect; that is, in other words, cures the disease.

Is not this law of cure, then, founded on nature, and does it not commend itself to our reason and common sense ? And when we see our remedies in small doses, prescribed according to this law, perform such wonderful cures, is it not just what we ought to expect ? We always know *why* we give any certain remedy, and know what its effects will be, for we have tried them in large doses on the healthy and understand their properties. How different it is with the Allopathic physician ! Let us see how he learns to treat a disease. He takes up, for example, the study of fever, with a view of preparing himself to treat it. He reads in his books that one physician recommends cold affusions, and another disagrees with him and thinks them dangerous. One advises wine and another insists that his patient should have only the most cooling drinks. Many prescribe Peruvian bark or quinine, and others object to these remedies as hurtful. Some recommend a free use of cathartics and others warn the young physician against their use. Some recommend opiates, others think them dangerous. And so on to the end of the chapter, almost every remedy in the *Materia Medica* being recommended by some and repudiated by others. Thus furnished, the physician goes forth to take the lives of the public in his hands, at full liberty, under high medical authority, to employ just what remedies he pleases, and sadly puzzled to make a choice. During all his practice he never has a glimpse of any law to guide him in his perilous work. The best reason he can give for prescribing any of his drugs is that somebody thinks he has found it useful, without knowing why, in cases that seem similar. It is an unmitigated system of guess work, and life-and-death experiment upon the sick and suffering.

How different it is with the Homœopath! When we see a patient with the symptoms of an ordinary attack of fever, we give *Gelseminum*, because we have taken it ourselves before hand, while in health, and know that it produces just that train of symptoms, and therefore *know* that it will *cure* them, and we are not disappointed. In another form of fever we give *Tartar emetic* for the same reason, and with the same result. We always know *why* we give a remedy, because we have a clear and unmistakable law to guide us.

We have constantly new diseases, or old diseases putting on new forms. We are prepared for them beforehand. Every Homœopathist knew, years before cholera appeared in this country, that *Camphor*, *Arsenicum* and *Veratum* would cure it, because these remedies have been proved on the healthy, and found to produce symptoms *like* those of cholera. And when cholera appeared, we treated it with the most triumphant success, from the very first; while Allopathic physicians were experimenting and their patients dying; and they are still experimenting on this and all other diseases. Even now, after so many years of experimenting, they cannot save half the proportion of patients that Homœopathists saved the very first year of its appearance. Is it strange that a man, with any feeling of humanity, should be anxious to diffuse a knowledge of a system of medicine possessing so many advantages, and so full of blessings to the sick ?

Finally, we feel certain that if the public mind can become imbued with the doctrine of Homœopathy, and generally adopt it in practice, it will be the most effectual remedy for the now all-prevalent and destructive quackery, and be a vast saving of health and life. Try it, and then decide on its merits.

	NAMES.	STRENGTH.	ABBREVIATIONS.
1	Aconitum napellus....	3rd in pellets...	Acon...........
2	Agaricus muscarius...	3rd in pellets...	Agar..... .....
3	Ambra grisea..........	6th in pellets....	Ambra..........
4	Ammonium carbonic...	3rd in liquid....	Ammon carb...
5	Apis mellifica.........	3rd in pellets ...	Apis...........
6	Arum triphyllum......	2nd in trit........	Arum ....
7	Arnica montana.	tincture.........	Arn...... .. ..
8	Arsenicum album	6th in pellets ..	Ars............
9	Atropine	6th in pellets....	Atrop ....
10	Belladonna...........	3rd in pellets....	Bell............
11	Bryonia alba......	3rd in pellets....	Bry ....
12	Calendula............	tincture. ..	Calend........
13	Calcarea carbonica....	9th in pellets ...	Calc...........
14	Cannabis sativa.......	3rd in pellets...	Cann...........
15	Cantharis........... ..	3rd in pellets....	Canth..........
16	Carbo vegetabilis.....	9th in trit.......	Carbo veg.....
17	Caulophyllin	3rd in trit.......	Cauloph........
18	Chamomilla.......	3rd in pellets....	Cham ....
19	China............	3rd in pellets....	Chin ....
20	Cina	3rd in pellets ...	Cina ....
21	Cocculus...............	3rd in pellets....	Cocc............
22	Coffea	3rd in pellets .	Coff............
23	Colocynth	3rd in pellets.	Coloc..........
24	Croton tiglium	3rd in pellets....	Croton ....
25	Cuprum metallicum...	9th in pellets ...	Cuprum ....
26	Drosera	3rd in pellets....	Dros ....
27	Dulcamara	3rd in pellets....	Dulc ....
28	Gelseminum............	tincture.........	Gels...........
29	Graphites.............	9th in pellets...	Graph..........
30	Hamamelis............	tincture...	Ham...........
31	Hepar sulphuris.......	9th in pellets....	Hepar..........
32	Hydrastis	tincture	Hyd...........
33	Ignatia...............	3rd in pellets ..	Ign............
34	Ipecacuanha	3rd in pellets....	Ipecac.........
35	Kali bichromicum....	2nd in trit......	Kali bichr......
36	Kali hydriodicum.....	3rd in pellets....	Kali hyd......
37	Leptandrin...........	3rd in trit.......	Lept ....
38	Macrotin	3rd in trit.......	Mac............
39	Mercurius corrosivus..	6th in pellets....	Merc. cor......
40	Mercurius iodatus....	3rd in trit.	Merc. iod......
41	Mercurius solubilis....	9th in pellets....	Merc. sol.......
42	Nux vomica...........	3rd in pellets....	Nux ....
43	Phosphorus............	4th in pellets....	Phos ....
44	Phosphoric acid.......	3rd in pellets....	Phos. ac.......
45	Podophyllin...........	3rd in trit.......	Pod............
46	Pulsatilla.............	3rd in pellets	Puls...... .....
47	Rhus toxicodendron..	3rd in pellets....	Rhus...........
48	Sepia	6th in pellets....	Sep.............
49	Spongia tosta...... ...	3rd in pellets....	Spongia........
50	Sulphur	6th in pellets....	Sulph..........
51	Tartar emetic.........	3rd in trit.......	Tart...........
52	Veratrum album.......	3rd in pellets....	Verat. ....

CASES OF 32 OF THE MOST IMPORTANT REMEDIES.

1 Aconitum nap.	17 Ipecac.
2 Ambra grisea.	18 Kali hyd.
3 Apis mel.	19 Leptandrin.
4 Arnica.	20 Macrotin.
5 Arsenicum.	21 Mercurius cor.
6 Belladonna.	22 Mercurius sol.
7 Bryonia.	23 Nux vomica.
8 Calcarea.	24 Phosphorus.
9 Caulophyllin.	25 Phosphoric acid.
10 Chamomilla.	26 Podophyllin.
11 Colocynth.	27 Pulsatilla.
12 Dulcamara.	28 Rhus tox.
13 Gelseminum.	29 Sulphur.
14 Hamamelis.	30 Spongia.
15 Hepar.	31 Tartar emetic.
16 Hydrastis.	32 Veratrum.

GENERAL DIRECTIONS.

The usual dose of pellets (size No. 3) for an adult is six; for children one or two, according to age. When the pellets are dissolved, which is preferable if pure water can be had, put ten or twelve into a gill of water, and give teaspoonful doses. When tincture of *Acon.* is used internally, two or three drops may be put in a gill of water; dose a teaspoonful. When grains of the triturations or powders are mentioned, what will lie upon a three cent coin (new style) may be considered about five grains.

The usual dose of a powder, when not otherwise directed, is two grains; or, if dissolved, three or four grains in a gill of water; dose, a teaspoonful. *Gels.* same as *Acon.*

When taking Homœopathic remedies, the patient must abstain from all other medicines, herb drinks, odors—as Camphor, Cologne, Hartshorn, etc—and avoid vinegar, pepper and spices; and, as far as possible, coffee and tobacco.

PRACTICAL HOMŒOPATHY

For the People.

FEVERS.

In a work like this, it would be worse than useless to treat of fevers under the various and numerous names by which they are called in medical books. We shall regard all fevers as one disease, with a number of varieties, and give the treatment for the principal different forms it assumes.

The great majority of fevers in this country are what they call Bilious, or Bilious remittent; because they give evidence of bilious disorder, or disordered action of the liver, and have a *remission*—that is, a period during which the fever is less—every twenty-four hours. This usually occurs in the morning.

This form of fever, after some days, or hours only, of languor, loss of appetite, and perhaps nausea, headache, and feeling of fatigue, makes its attack by a chill more or less severe, pain in the head, back and limbs, restlessness, a feeling of weakness, bad taste of the mouth and coated tongue. Its course will depend on the treatment. Under the physicking and drugging treatment, its course is generally prolonged for several weeks, and it often assumes, at a late stage, a low, typhoid form, and is not unfrequently fatal.

After the chilly stage is over, which may be from one or two, or six or eight hours, it is followed by dry heat, continued headache, restlessness, loss of appetite, more or less thirst, and a general feeling of severe sickness. The tongue becomes more coated with a dirty white, or yellowish color, the pulse is frequent, often from one hundred to one hundred and twenty in the minute. Toward morning, some remission comes on, and perhaps there is a slight moisture of the skin, the pains are less, and the patient sleeps more quietly. This is repeated from day to day. Sometimes the tongue is dry, and of a browner color in the middle. The edges and tips are sometimes red, and sometimes the whole surface of the tongue.

This form of fever, if well drugged, according to the usual Allopathic practice, as I said, is usually prolonged to several weeks. If *no medicine* is given—if the patient entirely abstains from food, and gratifies his thirst with water only, and if the surface is washed frequently, whenever the skin is hot and dry, and the room kept well aired, the fever will generally be ended in from seven to nine days. But under a good Homœopathic treatment, it is usually cured in twenty-four hours, and where this fails, in less than a week.

TREATMENT.—In the early, or chilly stage, put a few drops of *Gels.* in a tumbler, and add an equal number of spoonfuls of water, and give a spoonful every half hour till the chill ceases, and perspiration is procured, or the pain and fever subside. Then stop it as long as the improvement continues. As soon as the symptoms begin to return, renew it. In a majority cases, the first dose stops the chill within fifteen or twenty minutes. If the first dose produces no effect, increase it to two, three, or five drops, for there is a great difference in the quantity required by different persons. In many cases one-half or one-quarter drop is sufficient. After a free perspiration is thus produced, the pains subside and the patient goes to sleep, and when he wakes is conscious that his fever "is broken up." It is important that this treatment should be adopted in the early stage of the attack. I have cured innumerable cases by this remedy alone. This is applicable to all fevers that come on with chills and pains, as above described, whether catarrhal, (from colds,) bilious, typhoid or rheumatic. When these symptoms are present, *Gels.* is the remedy. If the treatment is not commenced till a later period, it will often succeed, and should be tried as the first remedy, but there is much less certainty of success. But it need not be continued over one day, if it is not obviously doing good. If this fails, and the fever puts on the forms and symptoms hereafter described, then corresponding remedies must be used.

Another form of fever comes on slowly and almost imperceptibly, without pain and with only a feeling of languor, or fatigue, and aversion to any effort. The mind is dull, and the tongue is either merely coated, or it is more or less red at the tip and edges, or it is dry and brownish through the middle. In such cases, f not soon relieved by *Gels.* give *Tartar emetic*, (four grains in a gill of water,) in teaspoonful doses every three hours, and continue it for some days. Under this there will generally be, after the first twenty-four hours, a daily abatement, and the fever will subside in a few days. If there is sleeplessness, delirium or headache, give, besides, a dose of *Bell.* three times a day.

In fevers, in which the bilious symptoms are most prominent, such as yellowish coat of the tongue, bitter taste, feeling of fullness or tenderness in the region of the liver, along the edges of the lower ribs of the right side and the pit of the stomach, costiveness, or bilious diarrhœa, high-colored urine, and feeling of nausea at the stomach, *Pod.* or *Bry.* and *Nux.* are the remedies. One may be given alone, or both alternately, three hours apart. If, however, the fever is high, and there is a good deal of pain in any internal organ, *Aconite* must be given, either alone or alternated with *Bry.* until these symptoms are subdued. And here is a good place to remark, that while *Gels.* is the best remedy known for simple fever, *Acon.* is the indispensable remedy for local inflammations, which often exist in fever. This distinction is of great importance, and should not be forgotten.

If the fever has assumed a low, typhoid character, with delirium, great weakness, dry lips, which, with the teeth, are covered with a dark crust, twitching of the tendons, and picking at the bed-clothes, give *Ars.* and *Bell.*, three hours apart. If there is a diarrhœa with this state, *Rhus.* is a good remedy. In children, *Merc. sol.*

Under this treatment very few fevers will continue a week. In the severe fevers it is of great importance to have fresh air passing frequently over the patient's bed, to carry off the effluviæ constantly arising from the body. It has long been observed in hospitals, that patients with fevers did not do so well when placed in a corner where a *current* of air could not pass over them. The whole surface should be sponged over several times a day with water of a temperature agreeable to the feeling. Once a day there may be a little saleratus or soda, or lye from ashes added to the water. During the continuance of the fever there should be a total abstinence from food, except water gruel, rice-water, barley-water, or similar things, made very thin, for a drink; and even these had better be omitted for several days, and only water given. The linen and bed-clothes should be changed daily. The patient should be kept entirely quiet, undisturbed by noise, and especially by conversation, and the room should be cool and not disagreeably light. After recovery commences, if the bowels are costive, give a dose of *Nux.* every night.

Intermittent Fever—Fever and Ague.

This disease is characterized by a succession of chills, fever and sweat, occurring very usually near the same time, or every second or third day. Between these paroxysms, the patient is comparatively comfortable, but never well.

TREATMENT.—During the chill and fever give *Acon.* or *Gels.* every two hours. During the intermission if there is coated tongue, impaired appetite and general feeling of illness, give *Bry.* and *Ipecac.* alternately, until the tongue becomes cleaner and the patient feels better. If there is not a decided improvement after two days, give *Ipecac.* and *Pod.* every three hours, or *Ipecac.* and *Nux.* for men and *Ipecac.* and *Puls.* for women and children. Within a few days, by this treatment, the disordered state during the intermission will improve, and the patient will feel tolerably well, except during the chill and fever. Then, if the chills continue, give *Ars.* every two or three hours.

If the chill comes on in the morning with nausea and vomiting, and severe pains in the bones, the *Eupatoreum perfoliation* or boneset is a very effective remedy. A weak infusion of the herb may be made and drank moderately during the day. In obstinate cases, *Polyporus pm.* tincture, five or six drops every three or four hours.

From thirty years observation and experience of Quinine, I am perfectly convinced that it has done infinitely more mischief than the ague would have done if left entirely to itself. It undoubtedly stops the chill and the fever temporarily; but these are only two symptoms of a general disease, which remains after the chills are stopped, with a more serious Quinine disease added to it. Thousands have thus "cured" an ague a dozen times in the course of a season, which, after all, still remains in an aggravated and more dangerous form than at first.

SCARLET FEVER.

There are three principal forms.

1—Scarlatina Simplex—Simple Scarlet Fever.

This comes on with many of the symptoms of other fevers. After a short time, the pulse becomes very quick—often, in children, 120 to 140 in the minute. The skin is hotter than in any other disease. The scarlet eruption comes out over the body on the second day, but may be seen in thickly scattered, red points over the tongue on the first day. The fever often produces delirium. There is usually some soreness of the throat. This is the simplest form of the disease and the mildest.

TREATMENT.—*Aconite* and *Bell.* are the chief remedies, alternated every two or three hours. Whenever the skin is very hot and dry, it should be frequently bathed all over with water at a temperature to suit the feeling of the patient. This if frequently done, in a remarkable degree diminishes the fever and quiets the nervous irritability. After a good bathing, the patient will recover from his delirium, become quiet and fall asleep, while the pulse falls from ten to twenty in the minute. I have practiced this free bathing in this disease, frequently with cold water, for forty years. The fear that it will make the eruption "strike in," is totally without foundation. A chill, should of course, be avoided.

2—Scarlatina Anginosa—Anginose Scarlet Fever.

This is a more severe form of the disease in which soreness and swelling of the throat is a prominent symptom. The throat is swollen inside and out. Swallowing is painful and difficult. If the inner surface of the throat is examined, it will be found red, inflamed, and often covered with a membrane, in patches of a dirty white, or ash, or yellowish color. The fever is high and the pulse quick. There is more prostration of strength than in the simple form, and more pains.

TREATMENT.—*Aconite* and *Bell.* are still the remedies in the early stage, alternated every hour or two. If ulcers appear in the throat, or if it is much swollen, omit the *Acon.* and give *Bell.* and *Merc. cor.* for men, *Merc. sol.* for women and children. If the throat remains ulcerated for some days, after the fever has somewhat subsided, omit these remedies and give *Hydr.* (ten drops in a gill of water,) in teaspoonful doses, every two or three hours, and gargle the throat after each dose, with a wash of the same, a teaspoonful to a gill. I have very recently seen the most beautiful effects from this use of *Hydr.* in cases where the throat is badly ulcerated. In obstinate cases, *Merc. iod.* may be preferable to other forms of Mercurius.

Scarlatina Maligna—Malignant Scarlet Fever.

This is a still more dangerous form of the disease. The prostration of strength is much greater, the pulse weak and quick—the throat dark red and ulcerated—there is extremely bad, fetid breath—the nostrils are often excoriated or raw with a fetid, acrid discharge, and there is a tendency to gangrene of the throat, and general sinking.

TREATMENT.—When these symptoms appear, give several doses of *Ammon. carb.* five drops in a gill of water, a teaspoonful every hour or two. This will frequently change the dark, threatening color of the throat, and other corresponding symptoms, in a short time. Follow this with *Hydr.* as above for a gargle, and give *Ars.* every two or three hours. Most of the cases, even of malignant scarlet fever, will be cured by this treatment. I need not say how hopeless they are with the common treatment.

The treatment given for this disease, in its malignant form, is equally applicable to the disease which has appeared in several parts of the country, under the name of the "black tongue," or malignant erysipelas. For dropsy that sometimes follows Scarlatina, *Ars.* and *Apis.* every two hours.

DIPHTHERIA.

This disease has some resemblance, in character and symptoms, to Malignant Scarlatina. From its late prevalence and its frequent fatality it is very important that its symptoms and treatment should be well understood. In its simplest forms, it usually comes on with chilliness, fever and languor. These symptoms are attended with redness, heat, and soreness of the throat, and more or less pain on swallowing.

TREATMENT.—When it appears only in this simple form, *Bell.* every two hours, is the appropriate remedy; or, if there is much feverish heat, alternate with *Acon.* If the throat is red and sore, a gargle of a teaspoonful of tincture of *Bell.* to a tumbler of water, after each dose of *Bell.*, has a charming effect. But if the disease goes on, there are soon other symptoms. There is more or less swelling of the throat, externally and internally, the nose is stopped, and discharges a thin or ropy mucus, the patient is more prostrate and languid, and complains of general soreness or lameness. When these symptoms occur, give *Bell.* and *Merc.* every hour or two.

But there is often sickness of the stomach, with pain and tenderness on pressure, great weakness, sweating or moist skin, with patches of false membrane over various parts of the throat, of an ash or straw color. Sometimes these patches are very small—mere points and few—sometimes numerous and large. With these symptoms there is fetid breath and often fetid discharge from the nose. In this condition *Am. carb.* is indispensable, three or four drops in a gill of water, a teaspoonful dose every hour, for five or six hours. Then if the membrane is not thrown off, *Merc.* and *Bell.* alternated every hour or two. When the glands are much swollen and the breath very fetid, *Chininum arsenicosum* as in malignant Scarlatina, may save the patient when other remedies fail. In these worst cases gargle the throat with *Hydr.* and if there is great prostration or diarrhœa give it as in Scarlatina. A recent successful treatment, for the false membrane in the throat, is *Kali bich.* and Merc. *iod.* in alternation every two hours.

There are other remedies often important, as *Nitric* and *Sulphuric Acid*, *Bromine* and *Iodine*, which are difficult to keep by families, for use. Indeed, this formidable disease should be in the hands of a physician whenever a competent one can be had. If the patient complains of heat and burning in the throat, there is no gargle so good as *Cayenne Pepper* in water, of considerable strength, every two or three hours, at the same time giving teaspoonful doses between, till the burning sensation ceases.

VARIOLA—SMALL POX.

This usually comes on with a chill, followed by high fever and severe pain in the head and back. In about three days the eruption appears as small red points, which gradually enlarge and fill with pus and finally assumes the form of a ring with a depression in the center which is characteristic of the small-pox pustule. These pustules dry up and form scabs.

TREATMENT.—

When the fever is high, give *Acon.* every two hours, for several doses, then *Bry.* to bring out the eruption. When the pustules begin to fill, give *Tart. em.* till they are pretty well dried up. This is probably the most important remedy in this disease. It moderates both the fever and the eruption and prevents pitting. Fresh air, frequent change of clothing and sponging well with warm water are very important.

VARIOLOID—MODIFIED SMALL POX.

This is an abortive form of Small Pox which occurs in persons who have been vacinated, and requires treatment on the same principles as Small Pox.

RUBEOLA—MEASLES.

This comes on with languor, a coarse, harsh cough, watery eyes, and fever, with pains in the limbs, headache, and chilliness. The eruption appears about the fourth day, but before this it may be seen on the roof of the mouth and throat.

TREATMENT.—

The remedy from the first is *Gels.*, but in smaller

doses than in fever, three drops in a tumbler of water, a teaspoonful every two or three hours, till the fever subsides. If the cough should remain troublesome, *Bry.*, *Puls.* or *Phos.*, every three or four hours.

The fever accompanying the measles cannot be at once "broken up," like other fevers, but can be greatly moderated during its course by *Gels.* and the eruption under its use is often but trifling. If there is troublesome, dry cough, or nausea, or diarrhœa, *Ipecac.*

VARICELLA–CHICKEN POX.

Is very much in appearance like Varioloid, but milder, and runs its course much quicker. The pustules being matured by the third day and dried up by the sixth day. In most cases no treatment is necessary. If there is some fever, *Acon.* may be given. If there is great restlessness, *Coff.* If the brain is affected, *Bell.*

ROSEOLA–ROSE-RASH.

This is an eruption of very small, bright red spots scattered over the body. There is generally but little if any fever, but it occasionally puts on a form resembling Scarlatina, attended with catarrhal symptoms.

TREATMENT.—If there is fever, a few doses of *Acon.* should be given followed by *Bell.*

URTICARIA—NETTLE RASH.

This is characterized by spots or wheels of various sizes over the body, generally white or a little red, and surrounded by a rose colored circle. It is a constitutional disease and requires general treatment. It is very commonly the result of indigestion produced by improper food. The attack is preceded by restlessness, oppression, want of appetite, and fever. When the eruption appears these symptoms are somewhat relieved, but there is a good deal of itching and sometimes swelling. The eruption sometimes suddenly disappears and the patient suffers from nausea, vomiting and fever. In this case *Bry.* is the proper remedy to restore the eruption.

ITCH.

Croton tig. and *Lobel.*, alternately, every six or eight hours, will generally moderate the itching in a single day, and, as I know, from experience, cure the disease in a week or two. If it fails after this length of time, or is not improving, give *Merc. cor.* three times a day for a week, and the first remedies, as before. Drying up the disease suddenly by external applications, is a dangerous practice, often producing a variety of internal disorders, and sometimes death.

If the disease is incorrigible, however, there is no danger in a weak sulphur ointment, (one part of sulphur to ten of lard,) thoroughly rubbed into the sores at the same time that *Sulphur*, in Homœopathic doses, is taken internally, three times a day.

ERYSIPELAS.

Consists in a diffused, and, at first bright, afterwards dark redness of the skin, with burning and fever. It appears in three forms; the simple, vesicular, and phlegmonous.

It often appears about the head and face, and is then a dangerous disease.

TREATMENT.—In the simple form, consisting of a simple diffused redness without great swelling, *Bell.* alone, or alternated with *Acon.*, is sufficient every two, three or four hours.

In the vesicular form, that is, where blisters rise on the inflamed skin, if it is on the head and face, *Bell.* and *Rhus.* If on other parts, the same, or *Rhus.* and *Graph.*, or *Hepar.*

In this form of Erysipelas, *Canth.* is a successful remedy, given in pellets every two or three hours, and a wash of the tincture, ten drops to a gill of water, applied to the parts which are to be kept wet with it.

In the phlegmonous form, that is, when the pain is deep seated, and the inflammation extends beyond the skin, in the parts beneath, with a good deal of swelling and severe pain, the two last remedies are good, but *Apis mel.* is probably the most reliable remedy. It may be given alone, or alternated with *Bell.* or *Rhus.* every two or three hours.

In all other forms of Erysipelas, an application of freshly-mashed cranberries will have an excellent effect.

RHEUMATISM.

Is characterized by pain or soreness or stiffness, affecting generally the joints or muscles, but sometimes the periosteum or bone sheath, or the pericardium or heart sheath. The inflammation frequently wanders from one point to another. The disease when acute is accompanied by an irregular fever and profuse sweats.

TREATMENT.—If it is attended with severe pain, redness and swelling and fever, especially if it comes on rather suddenly with chills, give *Gels.* By keeping up a perspiration with this for a short time, the disease will frequently be terminated. If not, give *Acon.* and *Bell.* alternately every two or three hours. When the inflammation has become somewhat diminished, give *Bry.* and *Colchicum* one drop alternately two hours.

When Rheumatism changes its place from one part to another, give *Bry.* and *Puls.*, two or three hours apart.

If there is profuse sweating, which does not relieve, but only weakens the patient, as sometimes occurs in this disease, give *Merc. cor.* for men, or *Merc. sol.* for women and children, every two or three hours, till this state is corrected.

This treatment will cure a majority of cases quicker than they usually are cured, but there are chronic and complicated cases of Rheumatism, which require skill and experience. If the disease has been long standing, electricity becomes an indispensable aid.

NEURALGIA— PAIN OF A NERVE.

The locality of this disease is very various, and wherever located, very distressing. One side of the face or head, is a very common location. It occurs most frequently in feeble and nervous females.

TREATMENT.—A majority of the cases will be promptly relieved by *Gels.*, but it sometimes requires to be given in pretty large doses, repeated every half hour till the pain is relieved. *Acon.* in drop doses of the tincture, and a wash of equal parts of the same and water, applied over the painful nerve, is often equally effectual; but if any feeling of numbness is produced, it should be at once stopped.

The disease usually consists of paroxysms with intervals of ease. During these intervals give *Ars.* every two or three hours.

If connected with disordered menstruation or female difficulties, *Mac.*, *Puls.* and *Sep.* during the intervals, only one at a time, every three or four hours.

CANKERED SORE MOUTH.

Give *Merc. Cor.* and wash with Hydrastis half every hour.

PHARYNGITIS—SIMPLE SORE THROAT.

In the first stage a few doses of *Gels.* will

often effect a speedy cure. If not, *Bell* and *Arum* or *Merc.* every two or three hours. If the throat becomes ulcerated, use a gargle of *Hydr.* frequently, as in scarlet fever, and give *Merc. iod.* or *Merc. sol.* If fever, *Acon.*

QUINSY—INFLAMMATION OF THE TONSILS.

In this disease the tonsils or glands of the throat, on one or both sides, are swollen, red, sore, and painful. The pain often extends to the ears. It is produced by a cold.

TREATMENT. *Acon.* and *Bell.* while there is much fever. If there is but little fever, *Bell.* and *Merc. iod.* If not soon improved, *Apis.* In those subject to the attacks of Quinsy, it will usually be avoided by washing the neck every morning with cold water, and rubbing it well and gargling the throat with the same.

PERITONITIS—INFLAMMATION OF THE BOWELS.

By this, we mean inflammation of the outer or peritoneal coat of the bowels. It usually comes on like other inflammatory diseases, with a chill. This is accompanied or followed by pain over some part or the whole of the abdomen, which is sharp and severe, often burning. The abdomen becomes sensitive and painful to the least pressure, and is more or less enlarged or swollen. A full breath is painful. There is often vomiting; the face is pale, and looks anxious and suffering. The breathing is short and quick, and the pulse quick and small; the disease is dangerous, and may be fatal in two or three days.

TREATMENT. During the early or chilly stage give *Gels.* as in fever, and keep up a perspiration for some time, till the pain and fever abate. But if this fails of giving some relief after a few hours, give *Acon.* and *Bell.* alternately every two hours till the violence of the disease abates; afterwards *Bell.* and *Merc.* every three or four hours. After the patient is fairly recovering, if there is constipation, give *Nux.* at bed time.

Throughout the disease, cloths wrung out of hot water, laid on the bowels and covered with flannel, and copious *hot* water injections greatly aid the cure.

HEPATITIS—INFLAMMATION OF THE LIVER.

This is known by pain just under the edges of the lower ribs of the right side and pit of the stomach, with tenderness on pressure. There is often a feeling of fullness in this region, pain on taking a deep breath, and a sympathetic pain in the right shoulder. If it proceeds very far there is obvious enlargement of the liver, producing a visible fullness in the region, constant dull or sharp pain, and a good deal of fever. There is a loss of appetite, perhaps nausea and bilious vomiting; the bowels are costive, or there is looseness, with discharges of unnatural color from unhealthy bile. The skin and eyes are often somewhat tinged with yellow. There is often a dry, hacking cough.

It frequently comes on with a chill.

TREATMENT.—In the early or chilly stage, *Gels.* is the most likely to "break up" the disease by copious perspiration. This remedy has the advantage of acting very quickly, so that if it fails, as it seldom does, not much time is lost. Two or three doses will determine whether the expected effect is to be realized, the dose repeated every half hour. If it produces perspiration, or abates the fever and pain, it should be continued as long as it does good.

If it fails, *Acon.* and *Bell.* may be given every two hours till the acuteness of the disease is abated. If some soreness and pain remain, the remedies are *Bell.*, *Merc.*, *Nux.*, *China*, *Pod.* and *Bry.*

Bell. is preferable if there is restlessness, fullness or pain of the head, fullness of the pit of the stomach, difficult breathing, thirst or dizziness; *Bryonia*, if there is a feeling of tightness, burning or stinging in the liver, more when pressing it, or when coughing or deep breathing.

Merc. if there is a yellowness of the skin, bitter taste, and tendency to chilliness.

Pod. for the same symptoms and irregular, loose state of the bowels, or nausea.

Nux. if there is considerable tenderness of the liver, thirst, red urine and constipation.

China applies to almost all the above symptoms, especially if there is considerable weakness. Either of these may be given every three or four hours.

COLDS.

Cold in the Head—Coryza, and Cold affecting the Bronchia—Bronchitis—Bronchial Catarrah—Cold on the Lungs.

TREATMENT.—If a cold affecting any of these parts comes on with a chill, or with a soreness or rawness of the throat, windpipe or bronchia, extending into the chest, or fever, *Gels.* is the prompt and sovereign remedy. A single dose will often "break up" the violence of the disease, remove the inflammation and soreness, and leave only a mild, loose cough, which will only require a few doses of ***Bry.*** or ***Puls.*** The patient with a cold at all severe should go to bed and keep quiet and warm till better. Medicine produces a vastly better effect when the patient is in bed, and keeps in a quiet and passive state, than when he is moving about.

If a cold is confined to the head, with stoppage of the nose, *Nux.* is the remedy every two or three hours till relieved.

If there is profuse, watery, or acrid discharge from the nose, *Kali hyd.* is perhaps the best remedy, but *Ars.* and *Merc. sol.* are effectual.

If there is a rough, raw, sore feeling of the throat or chest, with tightness, oppressed breathing and painful cough, *Gels.* is the remedy till these symptoms subside. *Kali hyd.* and *Phos.* are good remedies. When only a loose, painless cough remains, *Tart em.*, *Bry. Merc.*, or *Puls.*, will soon complete the cure. Abstain from food as in fever till the cold is relieved. If there is deep soreness of the chest, and fever, *Acon. Bry. Phos.* or *Tart. em.* are the best remedies. If catarrh has continued a long time, Cutler's Inhaler is the most certain remedy.

INFLUENZA

Is only an aggravated form of the above affection, prevailing periodically or epidemically.

TREATMENT.—Similar to the above—*Gels.* is the first remedy. If the symptoms are severe, *Ars.* and *Merc.* or *Kali. iod.*

PNEUMONIA—INFLAMMATION OF THE LUNGS.

This is distinguished from the preceding affection of the bronchia by the following symptoms:

It usually comes on with a chill, followed by high fever, a full, strong, quick pulse, short, difficult breathing, a *dull* pain in one side of the chest, generally the right, which prevents a full breath, white-coated tongue, and red cheeks. The pain in the side is sometimes changeable in its location for hours before it settles in one fixed place. There is cough from the first. The expectoration is, at first, white and viscid, or sticky and tough; at a later period it is reddish or rust colored. If there was doubt before, as to the nature of the disease there need be no longer, after this reddish expectoration appears, for this is a sure sign of inflammation of the lungs.

TREATMENT.—In the first or chilly stage of the disease, as in most other inflammatory diseases, *Gels.* is capable of breaking up the disease. If the disease has become established, the remedies are *Acon.*, *Bry.*, *Phos.*, *Tart. em.* and *Sulph.* I believe *Bry.* to be the nearest to a specific for Pneumonia. In many cases it is the only one needed. But if the fever is very high, and the pain and soreness great, give *Acon.* and *Bry.* alternately every two hours without change. *Phos.* may be given instead of *Acon.* if the fever is not excessive, if there is great weakness, bloody expectoration, or burning in the lungs. *Tart. em.* if there is great difficulty of breathing, gasping for air; if expectoration is delayed, or there is great rattling of mucus in the chest.

Sulph. if recovery is slow and difficult—a few doses.

PLEURISY—INFLAMMATION OF THE PLEURA.

This consists of inflammation of the covering membrane of the lungs. It has many of the general symptoms of Pneumonia, but the pain in the side is sharp, acute, stitching, instead of dull. It is impossible to take a full breath on account of this sharp pain. The pulse is sharper and smaller—there is less expectoration, and it is not bloody, unless it be some small *streaks* of blood. Not unfrequently the two diseases are combined, constituting what is called pleuro-pneumonia.

The same remedies are applicable as in Pneumonia.

NEPHRITIS—INFLAMMATION OF THE KIDNEYS.

This usually comes on like most inflammatory diseases, with a chill, accompanied or followed by pain in the back, (not in the spine, but on one or both sides of it; that is in the location of the kidneys,) tenderness on pressure in this region, fever, nausea, often vomiting, the urine scanty and high-colored, often bloody—the bowels constipated. The pain often extends down to the groin and neck of the bladder.

TREATMENT.—*Gels.* as in other inflammatory diseases, in the early stage, is the remedy, continued as long as it gives relief. This, if commenced early, "will break it up" by perspiration.

If this has been neglected, or if the disease has continued for some time, and *Gcls.* fails of producing the desired effect, and the pain shoots from the kidneys down to the bladder, and there is colicky pain, give *Bell.* every hour or two.

If there are shooting, tearing or cutting pains

with very scanty urine, which is passed with pain, *Canth.* every two or three hours. In general, these two remedies may be given to advantage, alternately.

During the treatment the bowels should be freely moved by copious injections of water, making a free use of warm hip-baths; that is, sitting in a tub of quite warm water, deep enough to come up over the hips.

CYSTITIS—INFLAMMATION OF THE BLADDER.

This comes on with the same general symptoms as the last disease, with pain in the bladder, constant desire to pass urine, which is very scanty at each discharge, often bloody, and passed with terrible pain, often with nausea and vomiting. There is a feeling of weight in the region of the bladder, and tenderness to pressure.

TREATMENT.—The treatment is nearly the same as that of Nephritis. If not soon relieved by *Gels.* give *Acon.* every hour till the fever is somewhat abated, and the most distressing symptoms somewhat moderated, then *Canth.*, every two or three hours.

MENINGITIS—INFLAMMATION OF THE BRAIN.

This disease is characterized by pain of the head, rolling the head from side to side, dilated or contracted pupils, throbbing of the arteries of the neck and temples, delirium, sometimes followed by drowsiness or stupor.

There is fever, with quick pulse. It is very apt to end in convulsions, when fatal.

TREATMENT.—The chief remedies are *Acon.*, *Bell.* and *Bry.* Give the two first alternately, every two hours, till the fever and other symptoms are somewhat abated; then *Bell.* and *Bry.* every three hours. Persevere in this treatment even though the improvement may not be very perceptible. Do not irritate and torment the patient with blisters, mustard plasters, or any other irritating applications. Shut out all strong light, avoid all noise, and especially conversation within hearing of the patient, (and the hearing is very acute in this disease;) keep the room well aired and of comfortably cool temperature, and disturb and excite the patient as little as possible. Do not apply cold water to the head. I have been entirely satisfied for years, that vastly more mischief than good is done by cold applications in this disease. Cloths wet in *hot* water may be now and then applied for a short time only, with benefit; keep the bowels free by injections of water, and keep the feet worm. Sponge over the surface of the body with worm water, if the patient is hot and restless.

In advanced stages, with dilated pupils, stupor, and other evidences of dropsy of the brain, *Helleborus*, *Merc.* and *Apis.* are necessary.

OPHTHALMIA—INFLAMMATION OF THE EYES.

SYMPTOMS.—Bright redness, pain and heat,

intolerance of light; dryness or watery, or thick discharge. If severe, with headache and fever and redness of the whole white of the eye.

TREATMENT.—*Acon.* every two hours, if there is deep redness and pain of a prickling, burning or smarting character, and profuse watery discharge. *Bell.*, when these symptoms are somewhat subdued and there exists redness, puffing of the eyes, aching pains in the eye-ball or orbit, pain on moving the eyes, &c.

Merc. after *Bell.* or when there are cutting pains or pain as from sand in the eyes, flow of tears, intollerance of light, pain in orbit or forehead, or inflammation of the iris or colored part of the eye.

Sulphur in very obstinate cases.

Never apply *cold* water or other *cold* wash to inflamed eyes. Hot water is the best application for acute, painful inflammation of the eyes.

Chronic Ophthalmia or inflammation of the eyes of long standing requires *Hepar.*, *Ars. Sulph.*, *Calc.* aud a different class of local applications, of which the physician can alone judge.

Cerebro-Spinal Meningitis—Spotted Fever.

This disease has become so prevalent and so fatal, that it is very important to be acquainted with its symptoms, so as to give it the earliest possible attention.

It usually comes on suddenly with a chill accompanied and followed by severe headache, pains in the back and limbs, and often vomiting.

Though the body is not usually very hot, the pulse is quick and the breathing rapid. Delirium, a tendency to throw the head backwards, squinting of the eyes, double vision and convulsions frequently follow. Often, but not always, the second or third day, red spots of various sizes appear on the body and limbs, which gives the disease the name of Spotted Fever.

TREATMENT.—A few doses of *Acon.* should usually commence the treatment, whether there is fever or not. Then a selection is to be made from *Bell.*, *Gels.*, *Ars*, *Bry.*, and *Rhus.* *Bell.* if the head is strongly affected, with delirium, flushed face, eyes red, with the pupils dilated or contracted, or convulsions, headache severe.

Gels. if the patient has a dull, stupid, intoxicated feeling of the head; dull, stupefying headache, dizziness, difficulty of keeping the eyes open, dim, blurred sight or double vision.

Ars. tenderness and pain in the nape of the neck, with stiffness and bruised feeling, dry tongue, foul discharge from the bowels and great weakness.

Bry., heat of the body which prevents sleep, but chilliness when uncovered, parts of the body on which one lies aches, violent headache, increasing intolerably by stooping, white or yellow coat of the tongue.

Opium, great drowsiness and stupor.

Cuprum may become an important

remedy in the paralysis and mental derangement which sometimes remains after the disease has subsided.

When the symptoms nearly equally indicate two of the above remedies, they may be given alternately.

STYE.

Puls., *Hepar.*, or, what is generally more certain, *Apis mel.* three times a day. Not unfrequently one or two doses will cure a stye when taken early.

CORNS.

Shave them close, and apply a little patch of cloth on which is placed a drop of the gum from the white pine. Let it remain till it comes off of itself, when the corn will have generally disappeared; if not, apply it again. This is a sovereign remedy. But this takes time. If the patient is in a hurry to get cured, touch the whole surface of the corn with strong Nitric acid, or Carbolic acid.

CHILBLAINS.

An application of *Arn. tinct.*, a teaspoonful to a gill of water, affords temporary relief, but internal remedies are necessary. Of these in ordinary cases *Agaricus* is one of the best.

If the parts become of a bluish red color, *Bell.*

If there is troublesome itching, *Nux*, and if a few doses do not relieve, *Sulph.*

If the parts are very painful, *Phos.* Any of these may be given every three or four hours till an improvement begins.

STINGS OF INSECTS, BEES, WASPS, ETC.

Ledum taken internally, and applied externally is a very effectual remedy for these stings, as well as the bites of musquitoes, flies, etc,, allaying the itching and pain in a few minutes.

I am indebted to Professor Hill for the information that a fresh onion applied to the part is a quick and effectual remedy. If applied immediately, it relieves in a few minutes; if later, it of course takes longer. A fresh piece should be applied ever ten or fifteen minutes. *Ammon. carb.* applied to the part, and taken internally often produces the same result.

BITES OF RATTLESNAKES, SPIDERS, ETC.

I have been for many years convinced from actual knowledge of many cases, that the most safe and effectual remedy is alcohol in any of its forms that can be most easily procured: as alcohol so much diluted as to render it tolerable, rum, whisky, gin or brandy. It should be taken in large doses, every fifteen or twenty minutes till the symptoms begin to abate, or the patient feels its effect. At the same time the part bitten should be kept wet with the same. It is surprising how large a quantity will be sometimes borne in these cases. A quart or two of strong brandy has been taken in an hour or two, without any other perceptible effect than to kill the poison and cure the patient. But the poison of alcohol proves quite a match for rattlesnake poison. It seems not to produce intoxication till enough has been taken to fully neutralize the poison, and the excess only produces the ordinary effects.

BURNS AND SCALDS.

Apply as quickly as possible, alcohol, whisky, rum, brandy, spirits turpentine or soft soap, lime water and linseed oil in equal parts or cosmoline, and keep it on, and keep the part thoroughly protected from the air till the pain subsides. Nothing is better than soft soap, and this is generally at hand. I have seen this applied from my early boyhood, and have never seen anything do better. Cold water though it feels comfortable for a moment is a very bad application. The above treatment cures burns in half the time. If there is fever, give *Acon.*

MECHANICAL INJURIES, BLOWS, FALLS, BRUISES, SPRAINS, ETC.

Arnica is the great remedy in these accidents. It should be taken internally in pellets, and the parts injured rubbed frequently, or kept wet with *Arn. tinct.*, a teaspoonful in half a pint of water. If inflammation and fever follow, give *Acon.*

But where the skin is broken, or the flesh torn, *Calendula* is the remedy, used externally the same as *Arn.* It acts like magic in allying pain and preventing inflammation, The edges of the cut or torn wounds should, of course, be brought as near together as possible, and kept there.

CARBUNCLE.

This appears, at first, much like a common boil, but larger and much more painful, and with much more constitutional disorder. It does not come to a point like a boil, but is broad and flat on the top, with several openings, instead of one. It is attended with chills, loss of appetite, depression of spirits, fever and prostration.

It more commonly appears on the back, or the neck. It is attended with great destruction of the flesh, which mortifies and falls out, leaving a large cavity which is very slow in healing. At the close the patient is as much reduced as after a long fever.

TREATMENT.—Give, in the beginning, *Ammon. carb.* three drops in a gill of water, teaspoonful doses every two hours, and apply a cloth wet in the same, (but twice as strong, and hot,) to the part—continue it as long as it does good. If it goes on, and openings appear in it, and the pain is not abated, stop this, and give *Ars.* every two or three hours. At the same time, apply *caustic* potash, powdered, in and around the openings, so that, as it dissolves, it will run into the openings, and penetrate as deep as possible into the heart of the tumor. Apply this once daily, placing over it a warm, soft poultice of slippery elm, flax seed, or bread.

The above treatment is much better and more successful than that ordinary practiced. The application of the caustic speedily changes and relieves the terrible burning pain of the carbuncle, and the *Ars.* aids in this, and preserves the system from running down, and greatly shortens the disease. Carbuncle should never be laid open by the knife.

MALIGNANT PUSTULE OR CARBUNCLE OF THE EXTREMITIES.

This affection is of frequent occurence during some seasons. It much resembles the ordinary carbuncle, but being located on the small extremities, it cannot acquire so great a size and is more rapid in its course. It seems at first, like the bite of some insect, and the patient generally thinks it is. It is at first a little red, somewhat pointed elevation like a small boil, with the appearence of a little hole in the tip. It is painful and burning. The inflammation increases rapidly, and runs up the limb. If it occurs on the toe, for example—the whole top of the foot becomes rapidly red and swollen.

If it goes on, it soon has several openings in it like a carbuncle, and ends in suppuration, and destruction of the substance, leaving a large opening. It is attended with a pretty severe, generally burning pain, and considerable feverish disturbance.

TREATMENT.—*Ammon. carb.* is the specific and effectual remedy, given as in carbuncle, and applied in the same way, The pain is often relieved in fifteen minutes, and in twenty-four hours the whole character of the disease is changed and the inflammation subdued. Since using this remedy, we have not found occasion for any other.

FELON—WHITLOW.

Apply as early as possible, strong Nitric acid or lye over the whole inflamed surface. If the application is painful, apply over it a warm poultice till the pain subsides. It not soon cured, lance it to the bottom.

For the last few years we have found a fresh lemon a sovereign remedy.

Cover the affected part of the finger with a slice of fresh lemon, and renew it every two or three hours. It gives immediate relief to the terrible pain and soon cures the disease.

AFFECTIONS OF THE STOMACH AND ABDOMEN.

CONSTIPATION.

A dose of *Nux* every night is often effectual. *Bry.* in hot weather. If it arise from torpid liver and want of bile, *Lep.* When very obstinate with very dry, hard fœces, *Plumbum.* Physic or laxatives in any form greatly increase this difficulty. A few doses of *Sulph.* is sometimes effectual, but diet should be greatly depended on for the cure of constipation. Avoid all high-seasoned food, stimulants and coffee;

live largely, and, if necessary, exclusively for a time, upon Indian mush, rye mush, Graham mush, cracked wheat, with syrup and a little cream, and ripe fruit, especially apples, figs, oranges and prunes. *Collinsonia* has proved an efficient remedy.

DIARRHŒA.

Under this head, we do not include the disease in infants. In ordinary cases, if it is produced by improper food, *Nux.* and *Ipecac* for men, and *Puls.* and *Ipecac* for women. A dose after each evacuation will be all that is necessary.

If the discharges are copious and watery, *Ars.* If not soon improved, *Ars.* and *Verat.*, or *Phos. acid.*

If the evacuations are bilious, yellow, green or dark, *Merc.* or *Pod.*, or both alternately.

If they contain undigested food, *Ars.* or *China*, or *Phos. Acid*, a dose in all cases, after each evacuation.

If the disease is at all bad, the patient should remain quiet in bed and abstain from food till cured.

If the disease has been of long standing, *Sulph* may sometimes be necessary. But generally it will be cured by *Ars.* or *Pod.* and *Lept.* alternately.

A patient who applied to me for a diarrhœa of two years standing, contracted in Panama, and who had paid over $500 to allopathic physicians without benefit, was cured with a small vial of *Ars.* When the disease has continued for a long time and the bowels are much weakened *Hydr.* is a very effectual remedy, in doses of one-half drop or one drop. Of late *Œnother*, a drop or two after each evacuation has proved an effectual remedy.

DYSENTERY.—BLOODY FLUX.

This consists in inflammation of the mucous membrane of the lower portion of the bowels, and is distinguished by slimy and bloody evacuation with pain and tenesmus or straining. without discharging any of the natural contents of the bowels.

TREATMENT.—The principal remedy is *Merc. cor.* after each evacuation. If pain extends over the bowels, or griping, give *Coloc.* alternately with *Merc. cor.* or *Ergeron Canadense.*

When this griping is alleviated, if there is no natural evacuation—only bloody mucus, or if there are passages of little round balls, give *Merc. cor* and *Nux.* If the disease has become established, do not be in a hurry to change this treatment, for it may require some days to effect a change.

If nausea and vomiting occur, give *Ipecac.* with *Merc. cor.*, or if there is much thirst with the nausea, *Ars.* till the sickness subsides.

An injection of warm water several times a day, does a great deal of good.

If, after a time, the evacuations become bilious, yellow, brown or dark, give *Pod* or *China.*

In dysentery of long standing, *Pod.* and *Lept.* alternately, are effectual remedies. Keep th patient in bed. If there is much blood in the evacuation, *Erigeron* is the most effectual remedy.

COLIC–STOMACH ACHE.

TREATMENT.—If this arises from indigestion or improper food, *Nux.* or *Puls.* If from cold drinks, ice cream, etc., *Ars.*

In *bilious* or wind colic with violent pain coming on in paroxysms, with disposition to bend forward, *Coloc.* in pretty large doses is a most prompt remedy, often curing the most violent colic almost instaneously. If necessary, it may be repeated in a few minutes. *Dioscorea* is equally good.

If there is great restlessness and bilious vomiting or diarrhœa, *Cham.* or *Pod.* In flatulent colic, or colic from wind, *Nux*, *Coloc.* *or Cham.*

SEA SICKNESS.

TREATMENT.—A dose of *Nux*, taken half an hour before going on board, will frequently prevent this for some time. When it is felt, *Nux Ipecac. Ars. Puls.*, and *Mac.* are very effectual remedies. One agrees better with some persons, and another with others. Armed with these remedies one need not suffer much from sea sickness. In obstinate cases *Petroleum* and *Silicea* are sometimes necessary, or *Cocculus.*

WORMS.

The three kinds of worms which usually inhabit the digestive canal are :

1st. Ascaris lumbricoides or long round worm. They are from 6 to 10 inches in length, and inhabit chiefly the intestines, but sometimes pass up into the stomach, mouth or nostrils. Symptoms : Occasional fever and pain in the bowels, starting in sleep, picking the nose, pale circle around the mouth, irregular appetite, etc. All of these symptoms however may arise from indigestion when there are no worms. The only reliable sign is the sight of the worm.

TREATMENT.—*Santonine*, third trit., every night, or what is equally good, *Cina* two or three times daily. But what are taken for worm symptoms are often the result of improper food, and are best cured by *Nux.*, *Puls.*, *Ipecac* or *Pod.* When fever attends worm symptoms, *Acon.*

2nd. Tenia solium—Tape Worm. These worms measure from 9 to 35 feet in length. Symptoms are more severe and persistent than those produced by the round worm, and are accompanied by the passage of segments of the worm about ¼ of an inch in length.

TREATMENT.—

Pumpkin seeds ground in a mortar to a pulp, in doses of two or three ounces, fasting, and followed in a few hours by a full dose of castor oil.

Kousso is a very certain and effectual remedy. Take half an ounce and steep in half pint of water, sweeten it, and give it all in divided doses during the day and evening, without any food. In the morning give an ounce of castor oil. This seldom fails to bring away the tape worm if there is one.

3rd. Oxyuris vermicularis — Pin worms. These worms inhabit the rectum or lower end of the bowels. They are slender and about an inch in length. Symptoms : Itching at the lower end of the bowels and the appearance of the worms in the stools.

Will be readily removed by *Merc. sol.*, a dose daily, and a daily injection of lime water. The lime water will not be made too strong if permitted to settle perfectly clear.

PILES—HEMORRHOIDS.

This disease consists in enlarged veins filled with blood, either within the bowel or just outside of the opening, or both. The tumors thus formed often become very painful, inflamed and tender.

TREATMENT.—If the tumors are external and very painful and sore, apply cloths wet in hot water. If not soon relieved, apply a tobacco poultice, warm. This, in the worst cases, will produce a temporary relief. If it produces any sickness, remove it at once. In the meantime give *Acon.* and *Bell.*, half an hour apart. Continue this external and internal treatment till the violent pain and soreness are abated.

The tumors should not be permitted to remain protruded externally, as it gives rise to great suffering and mischief. They should be oiled, and by careful pressure, returned entirely within the bowl, and secured there by a compress and bandage.

As constipation always increases the difficulty, the bowels must be kept in a healthy state. This is to be done by a regulated diet, brown bread, fruits, etc., and avoiding all stimulating drinks and highly seasoned food, and by approprite medicine. *Nux.* at night, and *Pod.* in the morning, will generally remove both the constipation and the tendency to piles. If not, *Nu*x. one night and *Sulph.* the next, continued for some time. I have cured cases of twenty years standing by this course. If there is burning, *Ars.*

In bleeding piles, if the bleeding is at all profuse, take *Phos.*, and if not relieved in a few hours, *Ham.* one drop every hour, and if necessary, injections of a gill of water and ten drops of the *Ham.*

Avoid physic in this disease. If necessary, it is infinitely better to use an occasional injection of water. *Lept.* is another excellent remedy in this disease, twice a day.

CHOLERA MORBUS.

This is characterized by an attack of vomiting

an d diarrhœa of bilious matter, with pain and cramp of the stomach and bowels. It is very distressing and may be dangerous, but is very quickly cured by Homœopathic treatment.

TREATMENT.—*Ipecac.* alone repeated every ten or fifteen minutes, is generally very quickly effectual. If the pain of the stomach and bowels is considerable, *Coloc.* may be alternated with *Ipecac.* This relieves the pain while *Ipecac.* stops the vomiting. If the patient has become much weakened, and the above does not promptly relieve, give *Ars.* and if the diarrhœa is at all obstinate, *Ars.* and *Verat.* alternately. *Iris.* is one of the best remedies.

ASIATIC CHOLERA.

In the commencement of the attack, a few doses of camphor, in doses of a drop, will often arrest it. If it does not, if vomiting is the most prominent symptom, *Ipecac.* every ten or fifteen minutes is often effectual.

But if there are copious rice-water evacuations from the bowels, and vomiting of the same, with thirst and prostration, the chief reliance is to be placed upon *Ars.* and *Verat.*, alternately every fifteen or twenty minutes. These are the only remedies generally required. If there are craps give *Cuprum* between the other doses.

Thousands have been cured by these few remedies by the peasantry of Europe, while from half to two-thirds of all cases were fatal under Allopathic treatment. It has everywhere been wonderfully successful.

JAUNDICE

Is marked by the yellowness of the skin and eyes, with languor, weakness, loss of appetite, coated tongue and often headache. The urine is high-colored and makes a yellow stain on the linen, and the evacuations from the bowels are a light clay color.

TREATMENT.—The remedies are *Lept.*, *Merc.*, *China.*, *Pod.*, *Nux.* Either of these may be taken separately, or any two of them alternately every three to six hours till improvement commences, (which will seldom exceed a few days,) then less frequently. By these remedies the disease is cured vastly quicker, and the system is left in a vastly better condition than under the old mercurial treatment.

This is a disordered state of the liver, which may be inflamed, for which see page 46.

BILIOUSNESS.

This is not a scientific term, but one which most persons understand. One feels languid, dull, sleepy, especially after dinner; he gets easily tired, his appetite gets impaired; often there is dull headache and tendency to constipation, and the complexion loses its freshness and becomes of a dirty appearance. People generally understand that these are bilious symptoms. They are not unfrequently the precursors of bilious fever or Jaundice.]

People having these symptoms generally suppose that they need a "cleaning out," and accordingly take bilious pills, or some other physic, which often results in a "fit of sickness." We can point out what all will find "a more excellent way," when they try it.

TREATMENT.—*Pod.* is generally the only necessary remedy. A single dose will often remove all these unpleasant feelings in a few days. If not, continue it three times a day in doses of a grain. If there is a tendency to chilliness or an inactive state of the bowels, after a day, take *Nux.* at night and *Pod.* in the morning. This course, for a short time, will save a fit of sickness and a doctors bill.

DYSPEPSIA–CHRONIC INDIGESTION.

The symptoms of dyspepsia are very numerous. Feeling of a load in the stomach after meals, sour eructation, heartburn, pain of the stomach, throwing up the food, dullness and pain of the head, low spirits, nervous symptoms, etc.

TREATMENT.—For the present relief from the effects of too hearty a meal, *Nux.* or *Puls.* every hour till relieved. For permanent effect —if there is constipation with other symptoms —*Nux.* before each meal, or for women *Puls.*

Iu ordinary cases either *Nux.*, *Puls.*, *Phos.* or *Pod.* before each meal will be appropriate. For heartburn, *Nux.* and *Ars.* alone, or in alter. nation with *Phos.*

A regulated diet, the avoidance of stimulating drinks and tonic medicines, bitters, etc., of highly seasoned food and physic, are indispensable.

One need not expect to be cured of dyspepsia by drugging.

In chronic cases, when the stomach has become very much weakened, the use of electricity will often expedite the cure in the most charming manner, and save months of treatment, or an entire failure.

Those of sedentary habits must abandon confinement, and take free exercise in the open air, daily.

Daily bathing with cold water, rubbing the surface well, especially over the stomach and bowels, is of great service.

In soreness of the stomach, heartburn, rising of sour fluid into the throat, and gulping of wind, there is no remedy so effectual as *Robinia.*

ASTHMA.

Confirmed asthma is a difficult disease to cure. The principal remedies are *Ars.* and *Ipecac.* Either of these may be given during a paroxysm every hour, till relieved. In nervous or hysterical women, *Acon.*, *Bell.*, *Ambra*, sometimes give relief. Distressing paroxysms are sometimes promptly relieved by sufficient doses of *Lobelia* to produce nausea. *Gels.* sometimes affords very prompt relief, especially if brought on by a cold.

But a change of climate or locality effects the

greatest number of cures. Many persons afflicted with Asthma at the East, are permanently relieved on moving to the West. Horses aflicted with the heaves—a similar disease—so as to be rendered useless at the East, are often entirely cured on being taken to the Western prairies. This is one of the diseases that is often most promptly relieved and eventually cured by electricity. Persons who have not been able to lie down for weeks, are sometimes able to do so from a single application. Cases which have resisted all other means are sometimes cured by Asafœtida in two or three grain doses.

COUGH.

This sometimes exists without obvious inflammation. *Bry.*, *Phos.*, *Balsam Cop.*, *Mac.* or *Arum* may be taken two or three times a day.

Hoarseness, without fever, will be removed by *Arum.*, *Spongia*, *Hepar.*, *Phos.*, *Kali hyd.* or *Nux.*

See the *Materia Medica*, in this volume, and compare the remedies.

A hacking cough is often produced by an elongated palate which requires removal.

PALPITATION OF THE HEART.

People who suffer from this affection are often frightened with apprehensions of heart disease. In a vast majority of cases it arises from other causes. We can only mention some of the more common causes and indicate the proper remedies.

From great loss of blood, *China*. From too great fullness of habit and excess of blood, *Acon.* From Anemia or pale, bloodless condition, often seen in young females, *Ferrum.*, *Calc.* and *Puls.* From nervous, hysterical temperament, *Cham.*, *Cocculus*, *Asafœtida*, *Coffea*, *Lach.*, *Puls.*, *Nux.*

From severe disappointment, *Acon.*, *Cham.*, *Ign.*, *Nux.*

From grief from loss of friends, *Ign.*

From fright, *Opium*, *Coff.*

From fear, *Verat.*

From excessive joy, *Coff.*

From indigestion or dyspepsia, the remedies for that disease.

From the drying up of eruptions or old ulcers *Ars.*, *Caust.*, *Lach.* or *Sulph.*

From disease of the heart it demands skillful medical treatment. When it cannot be had, *Cactus* is the most prudent and safe remedy.

BLEEDING FROM THE NOSE.

When this occurs after or during many diseases, as apoplexy, epilepsy, fevers, &c., it is salutary and should not be interfered with unless excessive.

If it occurs in pale persons, with scanty and thin blood, give *China.* or *Ferrum.*

If produced by a blow or contusion, *Arn.*

If it occurs frequently from slight causes, *Calc. carb.*, *Silicea*, or *Carbo. veg.*

If it is very profuse, *Acon.*, *Bell.* or *Arn.*

If it accompanies scanty menstruation, *Macrotin* or *Puls.* Hold both hands above the head.

BLEEDING FROM THE STOMACH—VOMITING OF BLOOD.

If there is fever, *Acon.* or *Bry.*, otherwise *Ipecac.* or *Nux. vom.* or *Erigeron Canadense.*

BLEEDING FROM THE LUNGS.

TREATMENT.—If there is much fever, *Acon.* every hour till moderated, then *Hamam.*, one drop every hour or half hour, or even one-fourth hour, according to urgency. If there is a sore, bruised feeling of the chest, *Arn.* is an appropriate remedy. If there is much weakness, with irritation of the lungs, *Phos. acid.*

ANGINA PECTORIS.

In an attack of this distressing affection, "the patient suddenly experiences, beneath the sternum, a feeling of strangulation and pain, which almost always shoots in the direction of the left arm, less frequently towards the right. This is accompanied by a distressing feeling of dread and sense of impending death. The sufferer imagines that he cannot breathe, but if forced to do so succeeds in making a deep inspiration. He does not dare to speak but groans and sighs. If the attack comes upon him while walking, he stands still seeking a support and clasping his breast. The hands are cool, the countenance pale, the features perturbed. After the lapse of a few minutes, or in a quarter or half an hour the paroxysm gradually abates, nearly always with eructations of gas.

TREATMENT.— Apply cold over the heart and warmth to the extremities.

In one of full habit, give *Aconite* frequently repeated.

If there is extreme difficulty of breathing, with pale face, feeble irregular pulse and fear of instant death, *Ars.* In extreme cases, camphor, brandy, or either in small doses may be of service. If these attacks continue to occur, and if connected with indigestion, *Nux* two or three times daily, or if attended with frequent palpitation of the heart, *Cactus* in the same manner may prevent the recurrence.

SYNCOPE—FAINTING.

This may arise from grief, fear and other strong mental emotions, going from cold air to a hot room, fatigue, fasting, breathing a vitiated atmosphere, loss of blood and other fluids, &c.

In any case the patient should be laid with the head low, in a current of fresh air, and if not quickly restored, sprinkle cold water in the face and hold camphor to the nose.

On a feeling of faintness, if there is palpitation of the heart or buzzing in the ears, *Acon.* If from loss of blood or other fluids, *China.* Avoid the causes enumerated above.

CANCER.

We do not mention this disease in a domestic work for the purpose of describing a treatment, but simply for the purpose of saying, that when anything of a cancerous nature is suspected, immediate advice should be sought from a skillful homœpathic physician. *Never go with such a case to a cancer doctor.* They never *cure* a *cancer*. They call every pimple and induration a cancer, and they sometimes get well after being converted into very ugly sores by bad treatment.

ENLARGEMENT OF THE GLANDS OF THE NECK, &c.

Frequently enlargements of the glands of the neck, especially in scrofulous children, continue for a long time and at last suppurate and discharge unhealthy matter.

In the early stage *Bell.*, *Rhus.* and *Merc.* are proper remedies.

If they continue long and threaten suppuration, *Hepar.*

After they have suppurated, *Silicea* and *Calcarea carb.*

GOITRE – SWELLED NECK.

This is a very common disease in particular localities, as at the foot of the Alps, &c. It has the characteristic slowness of scrofulous enlargements, and requires considerable time for its cure.

The following treatment will often effect a cure.

Take *Spongia* morning and evening, and rub the enlargement thoroughly once in three or four days with an ointment of *Biniodide of Mercury*, heating it with a hot shovel or smoothing iron. Do this at night and apply a flannel cloth round the neck, which may be removed in the morning. If this is not effecting a cure in two or three months, apply to a homœopathic physician.

POISONING.

When it is suspected that poison has been swallowed, give the patient immediately considerable quantities of the white of eggs beaten up with water or milk, then give an emetic of a tablespoonful of ground mustard. When the vomited matter becomes free from poison, administer a chemical antidote.

For acid poisons, common soda.

For alkaline poisons, as hartshorn or ley, vinegar.

For arsenic, hydrated per oxide of iron.

For lead, white lead, &c., epsom salts.

For copper, hydrated per oxide of iron.

For lunar caustic, (nitrate of silver,) common salt.

For opium, laudanum, &c., camphor.

For the secondary effects of poison consult the Materia Medica at the end of this work, and give the remedy which corresponds most nearly to the symptoms of the case.

HEADACHE.

Headache arises from a great variety of causes, and is attended by such a variety of complaints and constitutional conditions, that it is difficult to preseribe, except for individual cases. Each case is a study of itself. We can only give some general directions, which will, however, be found to apply to a great number of individual cases.

1st. It is often produced by indigestion or disordered stomach. This often goes under the name of sick headache.

TREATMENT.—*Nux.* will often promptly cure such cases if taken when the symptoms are first felt. *Pod.* and *Ipecac.* are often equally good; and for women, *Puls.* The same may be said of *Mac.* for women. *Nux.* at night and *Pod.* in the morning, will often prevent it in those subject to it.

2d. It often occurs in females as an essentially nervous disease, and is generally called nervous headache. In these cases, *Mac.*, *Puls.* and *Sepia* are frequently efficient remedies, and when relieved, an occasional dose of one or the other of these will prevent its recurrence.

If connected with female weakness, or accompanying monthly disorders, the last three remedies are specially applicable.

If connected with a hysterical state, *Mac.* or *Coculus.* If produced by grief, *Ignatia.* Either may be taken every hour or two till relief is obtained. A dose of *Mac.*, *Sep.* or *Puls.* daily, will often do much to prevent these attacks. But a remedy of extraordinary power, and which will cure a large proportion of what are called nervous and sick headaches, than perhaps any other, is *Atropine.* It is *most* applicable to those cases that are not caused by disordered stomach or other affection, but depend on a disordered condition of the nervous system itself; to cases that come on rather suddenly, and are very acute and severe. It may be taken every ten or fifteen minutes, till an effect is felt. Increase the dose if necessary. As soon as an effect is felt, suspend it till the effect ceases or while improvement continues. If an overdose increases the pain stop it altogether. When the temporary aggravation ceases it will be followed by an improvement.

This will cure a great number of habitual nervous headaches, which have resisted all treatment.

Those cases which come on with dizziness as the first symptoms, will be almost uniformly cured in this early stage by *Nux.*

In many cases of obstinate headaches, which resist all remedies, electricity, properly applied, is a most important remedy, but it must be applied by one who understands the human system, or it may do mischief rather than good.

I have effected many permanent cures of extremely obstinate cases by this means.

I have not given directions for the use of this powerful agent, because I have been long convinced, from many examples, that it cannot be profitably or even safely used by the public, at least without some experience, and special personal instructions. Nor is it a safe agent in Allopathic hands. It is a most beautiful and beneficent Homœopathic remedy, and to be either useful or safe must be used on Homœopathic principles and in corresponding doses. I have never had the opportunity of observing its use in Allopathic hands, when it was not, like other powerful remedies, in the same hands, as often productive of injury as benefit, and sometimes very serious injury.

FATIGUE.

When the muscles become fatigued by long walking, or excessive labor, or over exertion, a few doses, or even a single dose of *Arn.*, *Rhus* or *Gels.* affords great relief. If particular muscles by limbs are sore and lame, rub them with the *Arn.* wash.

DISEASES OF WOMEN.

AMENORRHŒA—ABSENCE OF THE MONTHLY TURNS.

When a stoppage or suppression occurs in young girls, *Puls.* three times a day, *Cauloph*, or *Mac.*, the last two alternately. If the menses do not make their appearance at the usual age, do nothing, unless the health suffer. In no case give what are are called "forcing medicines." They do great mischief, and are often dangerous, and are the source of long-lasting difficulties.

If sudden suppression is produced by a chill, or getting wet, put the patient in bed, give one or two doses of *Gels.*, put the feet in hot water, apply hot, wet cloths to the lower part of the abdomen, or use, if convenient, the warm sitz bath. If not soon relieved, give *Puls.*

If the suppression is produced by a fright, give one or more doses of *Acon.*, then *Puls.*

If, at the time when the menses should come on, there are nervous or hysterical symptoms, or spasms, *Cocculus* every hour or two.

If there is Leucorrhœa or whites, instead ot the regular menses, *Cauloph.*, *Mac.*, *Puls.* and *Sepia*, are the remedies—either one alone, or either two alternately, three or four times a day.

If suppression has been of long standing in girls, with paleness, weakness, palpitation of the heart, etc., the remedies are *Calc.*, *carb. Ferrum. Puls.*, *Sepia* and *Sulph.* Either of these may be taken three times a day for a week, when, if not improved, take another in the same manner.

DYSMENORRHŒA—PAINFUL MENSTRUATION.

If the flow is profuse with pain and sickness of the stomach, give *Ipecac.* every half hour till relieved. *Mac.* or *Cauloph.* may be used in the same way—the first especially, if there is headache.

If there are spasms in the abdomen, hysterical symptoms, difficulty of breathing, and especially if the discharge is black, *Cocc.*

For present relief, *Gels.* in five-drop doses is very effectual.

But *Cauloph.*, *Mac.* and *Puls.* are, in general, the three most important remedies. When there are no particular reasons for using other remedies the patient may take either of them, (perhaps usually *Cauloph.* is the best,) or either two of them alternately, every fifteen or twenty minutes, till the severe pain is relieved.

During the interval of a month, a dose of *Cauloph.* one day and *Mac.* the next will generally prevent these painful recurrences, and effect a permanent cure. But there are obstinate cases of this painful difficulty, depending on particular cases, which cannot be prescribed for without personal attention.

6

PROFUSE MENSTRUATION—FLOWING.

If this is attended with pressing down pains, and pain in the back, *Bell.* every half hour, till this is relieved. If much reduced by loss of blood, a few doses of *China.* But the most important remedy is *Hamamelis.* If at all urgent, a drop of tincture may be given every half hour, and if at all alarming, injections into the womb with a female syringe, if at hand, if not, with any other, of a teaspoonful of the tincture in a gill of cold water, and often repeated if necessary. This is equally appropriate, whether the flowing occurs at the monthly period or any other. All this is for present relief. But for those who have, habitually, too frequent and too profuse menstruation, and who are, at the same time, somewhat feeble, give, during the interval, *Nux.* every night, and *China* every morning for two weeks, and during the remainder of the interval, *Calc.carb.* one night, and *Sulph.* the next. This will seldom fail to bring about an improvement; but if this state is not entirely corrected, repeat the same during the next interval. This has cured many cases of long standing in one, two or three months, which have been treated for years without benefit.

The worst cases of *flowing* after *delivery*, are speedily checked by copious injections of cold water with *Hamamelis* or *Arn.*, and drop doses of *Hamam.* The cold water injections, so much feared by some at such times, are perfectly safe. I have used them hundreds of times, and for many years, and never had reason to regret their use.

PROLAPSUS UTERI, OR FALLING OF THE WOMB.

This is a very frequent and very troublesome difficulty, frequently imposing upon women long and painful disability. If a proper treatment is begun at an early period, it may often be cured by proper medicines. These are chiefly *Bell.*, *Calc. carb.*, *Nux* and *Pod.*

Homœopathic physicians have been strongly opposed to the use of mechanical supports, such as the numerous forms of pessaries and uterine supporters; and with good reason. Those hitherto in use have been very objectionable, producing great irritation, and entailing numerous evils, without effecting a permanent cure.

For the sake of the suffering, we are happy to say that a Uterine Supporter has recently been invented free from all the objections to former instruments. Experience has proved that with this improved Supporter, and proper medical treatment, instant relief is given, the patient is able at once to attend to active duties, and a permanent cure may be expected. It consists of an external padded abdominal supporter, to which a small ring pessary is attached by a silver wire stem. They are kept by Douglas & Sherman, Milwaukee, Halsey Bros. Chicago, and other Pharmacists.

We strongly recommend them in cases not readily cured by other means.

LEUCORRHŒA—WHITES.

This diseased condition, so common among feeble women, is seldom permanently cured by the old drugging process, astringents, etc., but the most stubborn cases are daily cured by skillful Homœopathic treatment. There are cases attended with ulcerations, and other diseased conditions, which require the personal attention of the physician; but by following the brief directions which follow, a great majority of the cases will be cured more promptly than is done by the ordinary prevalent medical treatment.

The remedies generally required in domestic practice are *Caul.*, *Mac.*, *Pod.*. and *Puls.* In most cases, the two first are sufficient. One may be taken every morning, and the other every evening, in a dose of one or two grains. Hundreds of cases will be cured by these remedies.

Pod. is especially appropriate where bearing down and Leucorrhœa come on after confinement—a grain three times a day.

If Leucorrhœa accompanies suppression of the menses, *Puls.* is the efficient remedy, three or four times daily.

When the discharge is acrid or irritating, or there is internal smarting, or burning, injections of the *Hydrastis* wash, as prepared for scarlet fever, is often extremely useful.

If the discharge is like jelly, or if it produces itching or burning, *Sepia* three or four times a day.

SICKNESS AND VOMITING DURING PREGNANCY.

This is sometimes a very troublesome and even dangerous affection, but by Homœopathic treatment can, almost uniformly, be promptly relieved. For this we have many remedies, and it is well to know several, as sometimes one agrees best, and sometimes another. Often a remedy gives prompt relief, but soon loses its influence, and another will be equally prompt. The patient may have the choice of the following:

Mac. in a majority of cases, is a sufficient remedy. If not, *Ipecac.*, *Arsenicum*, *Nux*, *Puls.*, *Sepia.*, *Pod.*, *Tartar em.* and *Verat.* may be employed, each with good effect in different cases. They may be taken from once to five or six times a day, according to necessity. A dose of *Mac.* at night, or *Ipecac.* etc., will often prevent the usual sickness in the morning.

CONFINEMENT—CHILD-BED DIFFICULTIES.

As a preparation for labor, a multitude of observing Homœopathic physicians now testify to the great benefit of *Mac.* and *Caul.* They render the labor much shorter, and much easier, and prevent after pains. Many who have always had tedious and difficult labor, have quick and easy ones, after this preparation. A grain of one may be taken at night, and a grain of the other in the morning, for some weeks before confinement. These two remedies have proved a blessing to thousands.

IRREGULAR AND INEFFECTUAL LABOR PAINS.

Caul., one grain every quarter or half hour till the pain becomes regular, which will generly be after one or two doses. *Bell.* and *Nux* are often effectual remedies. In tedious labors, from a rigid and unyielding state of the parts, *Gels.*, in doses of three drops, acts like a charm.

AFTER PAINS.

Caul. is the potent remedy, unless there is excessive flowing notwithstanding its use, when injections of cold water, with tinct. of *Hamam.* are required.

INFLAMMATION AND SWELLING OF THE BREAST.

Early in the attack, if it comes on with a chill, a few doses of *Gels.*, as in fever, by producing perspiration, dissipates the disease. But if this does not check the inflammation, give *Acon.* and *Bell.*, alternately every two hours till the inflammation is somewhat abated, and then *Bry.* and *Bell.* Keep the breast covered with a cloth wrung out of warm water. Do not permit the breast to become distended with milk.

But if the case has been neglected, or badly treated, till suppuration has taken place, and the breast is discharging, give *Phos.*, three times a day. If it has been of long standing, and the breast is very hard, after the discharging has continued for some time, *Calc. carb.*, *Silicea* or *Sulph.*, may be required.

SORE NIPPLES.

Apply, frequently, a wash of *Hydrastis*—ten drops to a tablespoonful of water. Or, if the nipple is raw, *Calendula* jelly. *Cosmoline* is a good remedy.

MILK-LEG.

Under the ordinary treatment, this is a most severe and protracted disease. The old school have never learned to *cure* it. The following directions will enable a husband to treat his wife for this serious affection, with vastly greater success, and cure her in one quarter of the time that is required by Allopathic treatment, in the hands of the most skillful physicians.

It generally makes its attacks within one or two weeks after confinement, like most other inflammatory diseases, with chilliness and fever. Pain usually commences in the loins, back and lower part of the bowels, extending to the groin, and thence down the limb. This commences to swell and in two days the whole limb may be twice its natural size. Though hot and inflamed, it is not red, but a very marked white. The feeling is hard and elastic. The disease consists of inflammation of the veins, and along the principal veins down the inside of the thigh and back of the leg, is the principal pain. These veins may be traced with the finger, enlarged and hard, like a cord, and very tender. These lines are interrupted now and then by a hard knob. Under the usual treatment, the limb does not turn to its natural state and size for a long time, often for years—sometimes never.

Treatment.—As soon as this affection is ascertained, give *Hamam.*, ten drops in a tumbler of water—teapoonful doses every two or three hours.

Rub the limb faithfully with a wash of the same—two spoonsful to a gill of water, applied as warm as possible. When the pain and tenderness are considerably abated, give the remedy less frequently, and apply it chiefly along the line of the hard and tender veins on the inside of the thigh and back of the leg by rubbing, and wet cloths. Continue this treatment less and less vigorously till the soreness and pain have entirely disappeared, and rub the limb with the wash daily, till the swelling subsides. If, after this, any considerable weakness is felt, give *Nux* at night, and *Ars.* in the morning. Under this treatment, this formidable and dreaded disease will be comparatively trifling. Dropsy will not follow this treatment. When it follows the old routine, its management is very difficult.

GENERAL DIRECTIONS DURING CONFINEMENT.

Never give physic after confinement. It is productive of infinite mischief. If the bowels are not moved in two or three days, give *Nux* at night and *Bry.* in the morning. If delayed four or five days, give injection of warm water this is always sufficient, and avoids the long train of evils that follows the use of cathartics.

The proper treatment of a woman, after confinement, is as follows: After resting for a few minutes, inject into the womb a pint of cool water, containing a few drops of *Arn.* or *Calend.* If the flowing is excessive, repeat the injection, using *Hamam.* instead. Apply cloths wrung out of cool water to the parts, instead of hot and dry ones. Wash the patient all over with a wet cloth or sponge, of a temperature to suit the feelings of the patient, with out too much exposure of the surface, and carefully avoiding any chilliness. After washing and rubbing dry, putting a wet bandage around her, instead of a dry one, covered with a flannel or cotton one, dry. Keep the room thoroughly aired and cool. Repeat the washing daily. Be no more afraid of water and air than before confinement. Under this treatment a woman will be as well and as strong at the end of four or five days, as two or three weeks, under the old abominable, physicking, confining and heating treatment. I am perfectly aware that many, both in and out of the profession, are horrified at this dreadful exposure at such a time. They seem to labor not only under a hydrophobia, but an airphobia. They relate cases in which women, after confinement, have been thrown into fevers, and had broken breasts, and even died from merely touching their hands to a cold wet cloth. This all may very well be. Shut a woman up in a tight, hot room, and roast her for several days, without a breath of fresh air, *before* confinement or *after*, and she will take cold at a very slight exposure, and so will a man. But let a woman go on after confinement with the same free use of both air and water, to which she has previously been accustomed, and she is in no danger of taking cold, unless the exposure is so great as to produce chilliness.

The advantages of the cold injections are the following:

1st. The internal organs, after labor, are hot, fatigued and exhausted. An application of cool water to them is always extremely grateful to the feeling of the patient, quieting and strengthening.

2d. It produces an immediate and prompt contraction of the womb, and thus insures the patient against an unnecessary or dangerous loss of blood, by flowing.

3d. It is a sovereign preventive of after-pains which often produce so much suffering and exhaustion.

This will be plain when it is understood how after-pains are produced. When the womb is not well contracted, but remains open, blood flows into it, and coagulates until it becomes accumulated in such a quantity that it excites the womb to contract, in order to expel it, just as it contracted to expel the child and afterbirth. The pains come on just as often as there is a sufficient accumulation of coagulated blood to render them necessary to remove it; no oftener. But if the womb is made to contract vigorously at first by a cool water injection, no such accumulation can take place, and there is no occasion for pains to expel it, and of course there are no pains. Why do after pains increase with every successive confinement, so that after a woman has had many children, they often become even more distressing than the labor itself?

It is simply because the womb becomes so much distended and weakened, that it does not contract promptly after delivery, but remains open, so that blood flows into it, in large quantities, causing repeated efforts to expel it, and each effort produces an after pain. A few injections of cool water, or cold if necessary, immediately, by giving tone to the weakened organ, produces the same prompt contraction that took place spontaneously in early labors, and of course the same freedom from after pains. I have witnessed the delightful results of this treatment for years, and in hundreds of cases. Many patients who had the greatest fears of it at first, are now loudest in its praise.

Hydropathic practitioners have long practiced it, and hundreds of other physicians, witnessing its safety and success, have adopted it, and *all* are delighted with it. I have received every year, from successive classes of medical students in the medical college, to whom I have taught the uses of water and air, numerous letters, thanking me for the teaching, and speaking in rapturous terms of the success of the practice, and the reputation they have gained by it. I have never yet known of the first case of mischief done by it, when administered with any sort of prudence. The old ruinous, roasting and physicking practice is fast going out of fashion, and common sense is taking its place.

The woman, after confinement, should abstain from all stimulating drinks, and have only light, unstimulating food, till after the milk is fully established. If the after pains require it, give *Caul.* By this course, the milk fever, on the second or third day, so common within my recollection, with often a broken breast in its train, will be avoided. A woman with a good physician and a good nurse, should have neither milk fever nor a broken breast.

NURSING SORE MOUTH.

This is a sore mouth mostly affecting nursing women, but sometimes coming on some weeks before confinement. Under the old treatment, it is very troublesome and often an incorrigible disease. If it continues for some time, it frequently extends along the mucous membrane of the stomach and bowels, producing intolerance of food, and an obstinate diarrhœa, under which the patient is rapidly exhausted. Many mothers are obliged to wean the child before the disease can be cured.

By a very simple Homœopathic treatment, it is almost invariably and rapidly cured.

TREATMENT.—*Pod.*, three grains in a tumbler of water, a teaspoonful before each meal, and at bedtime, if begun in an early stage, often effects a speedy cure. If the case is not improving in a few days, take *Nux* every night, and *Ars.* every morning. I have cured cases with these two remedies in a week or ten days, that had been six or eight months under treatment without benefit.

Hydrastis is in many cases, an invaluable remedy, every three or six hours. It may be made of the strength of six or eight drops to a tumbler of water, and taken in teaspoonful doses; the mouth being well washed with the same, before each dose, or the wash may be made two or three times as strong.

In cases of long standing, where the bowels have become affected, and the above treatment is not successful after a reasonable trial *Pod.* and *Lept.* are invaluable. One may be taken at a time, or the two alternated, every three or six hours—two or three grains, in half a tumbler of water, and teaspoonful doses.

There is not one case of nursing sore mouth in a hundred that will not be cured by this treatment, and in a much shorter time than it is usually done under medical supervision.

In a few obstinate cases, in diseased constitutions, it may be necessary to take *Sulph.*, two doses daily, for a few days, or *Sulph.* and *Calc. carb.*

A weak solution of *Carbolic acid* as a wash for the mouth is excellent.

NERVOUSNESS.

Many women, as well as some men, in bad health, have a train of symptoms well known as nervous. These symptoms generally depend upon a diseased or disorded state of some organ or organs, of which this nervous condition is only a symptom, and which must be cured in order to remove this symptom. But these distressing nervous sensations may often be greatly alleviated by palliative remedies. One of the most generally useful is *Ambra grisea*. In almost any condition attended with nervous restlessness, and sleeplessness, if not in acute fever, or inflammation, an occasional dose of *Ambra* will allay the irritability, and procure sleep, without any of the disagreeable consequences of opiates.

Coffea., *Acon.*, *Bell.*, *Cham.*, *Ign.* *Nux* and *Puls.*, often allay nervous irritability.

MILK FEVER.

(See General Direction during Confinement.)

DISEASES OF CHILDREN.

THRUSH.

This white, flaky eruption in the mouth of children is familiar to all. The mouth is sore and nursing is painful. There is no better remedy than *Borax* dissolved in water and applied several times daily over the mouth, with a soft swab. The child will swallow enough for an internal remedy. At the same time *Cham.* may be given, alternated with *Merc. sol.*, each twice daily. If it is obstinate, instead of *Merc.* give *Sulphur.*

SORE MOUTHS OF INFANTS.

Touch the mouth all over the sore surface, not rub it, with a wash of *Hydrastis* of the strength of ten drops to a tablespoonful of water, three or four times a day. The child will swallow a sufficient quantity for a dose each time it is used. *Merc.*, *Nux*, *Cham.* and *Sulph. acid*, are also effectual remedies. Either of them may be given three or four times a day.

STOPPAGE OF THE NOSE—CATARRH—SNUFFLES.

Nux is the sufficient remedy. Besides giving it internally three or four times a day, a prompt method of relief is, to rub a few pellets very fine with a little sugar, and blow a few grains up the nostrils through a quill. *Sambucus* is a good remedy.

CRYING.

When infants cry, it is always for some good reason. Endeavor carefully to ascertain the cause. It may be an uncomfortable state of the dress. It may be chafed, and the sore parts are rendered painful by being suffered to remain wet. It may be earache, or more probably, colic. If it is chafed, keep the parts dry—give *Cham.* three times a day, and wash the parts as often with *Hydrastis* as for sore mouth; or *Calendula.* If not soon better, give *Sulph.* twice a day. If it proceeds from earache, the child will manifest it by uneasy movements of the head, and often by screams. In this case, if there is fever, give *Acon.* and *Bell.* every two hours, till the fever subsides, then *Bell.* alone. If this fails, after a few doses, give *Cham.* and *Puls.* If the crying arises from colic, give *Cham.*, *Coloc.* or *Bell.*

A great deal of colicky pain and crying are caused by feeding the child when it should not be fed. It is a mistaken and very mischievous notion, that a child must have food within a few hours after birth. If this were so, an Allwise Creator, who makes all necessary provision for His creatures, would have provided it. The bare fact that the mother does not usually have milk for it before the second or third day, is sufficient proof that the child does not need it before that time. For at least thirty-six hours it should not be fed at all, unless the mother furnishes food before. A teaspoonful of water occasionally is the only thing it should swallow.

Above all, avoid medicine of every description even catnip or saffron tea. Some seem to suppose that every child is sick or starving as soon as it draws its first breath, and it must be outraged by unnatural food, and more unnatural medicine. Nine-tenths of all the fits, the vomiting, the colic and the crying, in young children, are produced by this abominable and unnatural treatment. Dr. Dewees, whose experience is very great, says he has never known a young infant to have fits that had not been fed or dosed.

If the mother's milk, from any cause is delayed longer than thirty-six hours, the child may be cautiously fed with a mixture of new thin cream, from milk that has stood not more than two or three hours, and water, with the slightest perceptible taste of pure, white sugar; the proportion being three parts of water to one of cream.

SUMMER COMPLAINT.

There are two distinct diseases that go by this name, viz: Cholera Infantum and Diarrhœa. The most obvious distinction between them is, that the first is attended with vomiting, and the latter is not.

CHOLERA INFANTUM.

This is a very prevalent and very fatal disease in this country, especially in cities. It chiefly affects children between the ages of three months and three years. It sometimes comes on with vomiting and diarrhœa at the same time, but quite as often the vomiting does not come on till the diarrhœa has continued for a few hours, or a day or two. It is often rapid in its progress, and fatal in two or three days. At other times it is of long continuance, and reduces the little sufferer to a skeleton. It is attended with considerable fever, coated or red tongue, quick pulse, a good deal of pain and suffering, great restlessness, and rapid failure of strength. The child sleeps with the eyes partly open. The evacuations are frequent, and exceedingly various in appearance, being yellow, brown, or green—often grass-green, or mixed, and sometimes the color often changing, scarcely any two evacuations being alike. In this disease, there is always inflammation of the mucous membrane of the stomach, or bowels, or both, and inflammation and congestion of the liver. Vomiting or diarrhœa will predominate according as the stomach or bowels, are most effected. If the disease goes on for some time, the brain is apt to become sympathetically affecte d, and under the Allopathic treatment of opiates, hopelessly diseased.

TREATMENT.—In the early part of vomiting and diarrhœa, give *Ipecac.* after every act of vomiting or purging. This alone is often sufficient to arrest the disease. If it fails, and especially if there is thirst, give *Ars.* in the same manner, not more than four pellets in half a tumbler of water, teaspoonful doses. If there is great restlessness, *Cham.*, alternated with either of the above remedies.

If the evacuations are yellow, brown or dark, *Pod.* is an effectual remedy; two grains in a tumbler of water, a teaspoonful, same as other remedies. When the evacuations are green *Agar.* is the best remedy, or *Cham.*, *Merc. sol.* or *Pod.*

If the patient is much reduced, and vomiting and diarrhœa continues, *Ars.* and *Verat.*

In many obstinate and protracted cases, when there is reason to believe that the bowels are ulcerated, *Hydras.* will save the patient.

Pod., in alternation with either of the above two remedies, is also applicable in the same case.

DIARRHŒA.

Occuring in hot weather, or from indigestion, is usually quickly arrested by *Ipecac.* or *Nux*, or both alternated. If the evacuations are thin and watery, *Ars.* alone or with *Verat.*

If they are green, *Agar.*, *Ham.* or *Merc.* If they are yellow, brown or dark, *Pod.*

If the disease has been of long standing, *Pod.* and *Lept.* or *Hydras.*, will often effect cures in cases that seem very discouraging. The remedy should be repeated after each evacuation.

There is no disease which requires greater caution in diet than Cholera Infantum and Diarrhœa. When cases are almost cured, the least imprudence in diet will cause a relapse, which may be fatal. *Dulc.* is sufficient in a great many cases of Diarrhœa, especially in damp weather.

INCONTINENCE OF URINE—WETTING THE BED.

The principal remedies are *Apis. mel.*, *Canth.* and *Pod.* One of them may be given three or four times a day. *Phos. acid* is often effectual.

CONVULSIONS—SPASMS—FITS.

These are frequently produced by indigestible food, or excess, as from raisins, nuts, pastry, etc. In these cases, if it can be done, get down a sufficient quantity of warm water to produce vomiting. Whether this is effected or not, give *Nux*, two or three doses, every two or three hours.

If from worms, *Santonine* or *Cina*, as directed under that head. If from a nervous condition, without the above obvious causes, *Bell.*, *Cham.*, *Ambra*, *Nux*, or *Ignatia*.

During the fit put the child in a cold bath, and apply the cloth wet in cold water to the head, then wrap in warm flannels, and get the patient warm as soon as possible.

RICKETS—WEAKNESS OF THE LIMBS—SLOWNESS IN LEARNING TO WALK.

This disease has a good deal of resemblance to some forms of Scrofula. It usually occurs during or before the first set of teeth. It is characterized by slow formation, softness and weakness of the bones.

The fontanelle or open place on the top and front of the skull remains open. The child is weak, averse to motion and looks sickly. The teeth are slow in coming, the long bones of the legs and arms are soft and can be considerably bent. The muscles are weak, the child has difficulty in holding up its head and has not strength to walk. The arms and legs are small and the belly large. There is often diarrhœa.

Homœopathic treatment makes one of its greatest triumphs in this disease.

TREATMENT.—The all-sufficient remedies are *Calc. carb.*, *Phosphorus*, *Silicea* and *Sulphur*; of these, *Calc.* is the most important, and one dose a day may be given for a week and then omit a week or more, and then repeat or give one of the other remedies in the same manner for a week, and so on.

Consult the Materia Medica for a choice.

The child should not be urged to exert itself when it complains of motion, nor should it be much in sitting posture, as the bones are liable to become crooked. To avoid this it is better to be lying than sitting, or attempting to stand.

It should be as much as possible in the open air, and be bathed in as cool water as can be comfortably borne, and thoroughly rubbed daily.

A change will soon be evident and a cure eventually effected.

SCROFULA.

Scrofulous affections occur in two forms, the acute and the chronic. The acute or tuberculous form is accompanied by persistent fever, emaciation and the deposit of a peculiar cheese-like substance called tubercle. The deposit may take place in almost any organ of the body. When it is formed in the lungs it constitutes the dreadful scourge of our race, consumption.

The chronic form of scrofula is characterized by slow and gradual enlargements and suppuration of the lymphatic glands, inflammation of the eyes, persistent catrrrh, thickening of the upper lip and pustular eruptions on the skin.

The one prominent feature is defective nutrition.

TREATMENT.—Nourishing diet, fresh air, out-door exercise and regular habits are as important as proper medication. Where there is emaciation, *cod liver oil* is a valuable aid to nutrition. The most important remedies are *Sulph.*, *Calc. carb.*, *Kali hyd.*, *Phos.* and *Sil.*, in the chronic or glandular form; and *Acon.*, *Bell.* and *Ars.* in the acute or tubercular form.

Consult Materia Medica.

CROUP.

There are two forms of croup, differing widely in their nature, and requiring an entirely different treatment.

Spasmodic or False Croup, is much the more

common. It comes on suddenly, almost always in the night; with noisy, wheezing, difficult breathing, sometimes threatening suffocation, sometimes with and sometimes without fever. This form of croup is usually quickly cured by *Acon.* and *Spongia.*

Membranous Croup. much the more dangerous, comes on more gradually, and more like a cold; with chilliness, sneezing, some soreness of the throat, hot skin, hoarse voice, and more or less difficulty of breathing. The fever, difficult breathing, with croupy, ringing sound, and other alarming symptoms, gradually increase, till suffocation is imminent. In this form *Kali bichr.*, *Hepar*, *Spongia*, *Tartar emetic* and *Sulph. acid* are the remedies to be depended upon. *Acon.* may be occasionally given, to diminish fever, but it can do nothing to prevent or remove the false membrane that is threatening to fill up the air passages, and produce suffocation. *Kali bichr.* is perhaps the most important. It may be alternated with *Hepar* or *Spongia.* If it does not succeed, *Sulph. acid* is the next most reliable. This should be put in water, and made strong enough to taste acid, and given every hour. Desperate cases are sometimes cured by it.

At the beginning, put a cloth wrung out of cold water over the throat and chest, and cover it well with a flannel; renew every hour.

WHOOPING COUGH.

The remedies most frequently required in the early stage are *Bell.* and *Nux* alternately, a dose after each paroxysm of cough. If there is fever, *Aconite*. If without fever, the paroxysms are very violent with nose-bleed, *Drosera*. If the chest is stuffed, and breathing difficult, *Tartar emetic*. If the chest is sore and coughing painful *Arnica*, *Bromide of Ammonium*, if the cough is frequent and severe and the patient's sleep is disturbed, gives relief. If the paroxysms are very severe, with tendency to spasms, *Cuprum* is needed. The patient should eat and drink sparingly, as a full stomach is sure to bring on a paroxysm of coughing. Exercise should be very moderate as well as talking or anything that increases the breathing. Avoid sudden changes of temperature.

MUMPS.

Most persons know this disease of childhood as a swelling of the glands just below the ear, and often extending considerably so as to give the sides of the face and neck a very full appearance.

Mercurius sol. is generally the only neccessary remedy. Avoid exposures of the face to cold. If exposed to cold, the swelling is liable to leave the face and locate itself upon other glands or organs. where it may be much more serious.

FALLING OR PROTRUSION OF THE BOWELS.

Nux and *Ignatia* are the best remedies, but only one at a time, three or four times a day, or *Aesculus*.

TEETHING.

The process of cutting teeth often produces great disturbance in the infantile organism. The child is feverish, and often exceedingly peevish and irritable. *Acon.* and *Gels.* are effective remedies while there is a feverish state, repeated as often as required. If there is no fever, *Ambra* or *Coffea.*

When there is dullness, and stupor, *Gels.* is the remedy.

INFLAMMATION OF THE EYES.

Is attended by redness of the lids, extending to the ball, swelling of the lids, aversion to light, discharge of matter, which sticks the lids together. In bad cases, ulceration of the cornea quickly follows, and the eye may be destroyed if not early and well treated. *Acon.* is the best remedy at first. If not yielding in a day or two, and there is much discharge, *Merc. sol.* If the light is very painful, *Cham.* or *Bell.* If the child is scrofulous, consult *Calcarea* and *Sulphur* in the Materia Medica at the end of the book.

SCURF ON THE HEAD.

Avoid irritating it by combing, and give one dose of *Sulphur* daily.

CRUSTA LACTEA—MILK CRUST.

If there is feverishness, give *Acon.*, till it subsides. Then *Rhus* three times daily for a week.

Juglans after this is usually an effective remedy—*Sepia*, is regarded by some as almost a specific. *Lappa major* is now thought to be a good remedy. *Viola tric.* is highly esteemed.

If the crusts become thick and hard, apply a bran, flax-seed or slippery elm poultice till they become softened and then carefully remove them, so as not to leave a bleeding surface. Wash the head occasionally with warm water and fine Castile soap, avoid all drying ointments and washes. If the disease is unusally obstinate, the use of sulpher twice a day for a week may be required.

MATERIA MEDICA.

CHARACTERISTIC INDICATIONS FOR MANY OF THE MORE FREQUENTLY REQUIRED MEDICINES.

ACONITE.

Chilliness and shivering. Shooting and acute pains; worse at night. Great internal heat, even with chilliness. General heat of the body, with pains of the head, back and limbs. Skin dry and burning. Restless sleeplessness, with tossing trom side to side. Starting in sleep.

Congestions of all the organs, external and internal, with low pulse and chilliness, and succeeding inflammation, with heat, pain, and high pulse. Dryness of mouth and tongue.

Watery diarrhœa, with white stools, and red urine.

Short, dry cough, with tickling in the throat, heat, thirst, and difficult breathing.

Palpitation of the heart, with great anguish. Very painful neuralgia.

AGARICUS.

Itching, burning, and redness of the fingers and toes, and other parts, as from frost-bite.

Dizziness and headache, as from intoxication. Painful sensitiveness of the scalp.

Chapping of the upper lip. Palpitation of the

heart when standing. Profuse sweat on the chest at night.

AMBRA GRISEA.

Nervousness, with great irritability of temper.

Great languor in the morning in bed. Drowsiness during the day; restless sleeplessness during the whole night, and weariness in the morning.

Low spirits and extreme nervousness.

Painful spot on the top of the head.

The hair feels sore, when touched.

The arms go to sleep easily.

Cramps in the hands and legs.

Burning in the bottoms of the feet.

AMMONIUM CARBONICUM.

Boils and pustules on the nose and face. Freckles. Face pale and bloated. Burning vesicles on the inside of the lips and tongue. Burning on the tip of the tongue, painful to the touch.

Sore throat, which is very dark red, or black, with fetid breath.

Obstinate nursing sore mouth.

Violent, acrid leucorrhœa, causing soreness. Watery, burning leucorrhœa.

APIS.

Chronic headache, in nervous subjects, which is moderated by pressure.

Inflammation of the peritoneum, or outer coat of the intestines, characterised by burning, internal soreness, and external tenderness, even on slight pressure. Abdomen full, swollen, tender.

Dropsy, especially after scarlet fever. Dropsy of the abdomen and brain.

Nettle rash, and other itching, stinging, pricking and burning eruptions. Stye.

ARUM TRIPHYLLUM.

Cold with irritation of the eyes nose and throat. Nose stopped or discharging an acrid fluid.

Sore tongue, mouth and throat, with biting, stinging pain. Tickling burning in the throat.

ARNICA.

Mechanical injuries, as falls, blows, sprains, bruises and concussions.

Pains in the limbs as if bruised.

Burning in the brain, the rest of the body being cool. Headache, increased by stooping, with heat of the head and face.

Pain in the back, as if bruised and lame.

A succession of small boils.

ARSENICUM.

Rapid sinking of strength; feels stronger on lying down, but weak on standing. Fainting fits. Great emaciation of children.

General dropsy. Dropsy after scarlet fever. Intermittent fever, with violent chills, increased by drinking, and in the open air; the heat, dry, and burning, followed by scanty or cold, clammy sweats.

Religious melancholy. Violent *periodical* headache, relieved by the application of cold water.

The hair is painful and sore.

Inflammation of the eyes, with *burning* pain.

Sunken, pale face, or livid and blue. Puffed, bloated face. Bluish lips.

In fevers, tongue bluish or white; or red and dry; or brown and blackish.

Burning inflammation of the throat. Throat dark red, with fetid breath.

Violent vomiting of yellow-green mucus and bile; of brownish or blackish substance. During the vomiting, violent pain in the stomach. Vomiting and diarrhœa. Cholera morbus. Asiatic cholera. Pain of the abdomen, with vomiting and diarrhœa. Violent diarrhœa, with colic. Vomiting and great weakness. Piles, *burning* and painful.

Colds, with watery discharge from the nose; sneezing, or dryness of the nose; scraping of the throat, with soreness; hoarseness; short, hacking cough, with soreness of the chest; sense of suffocation and anxious, short breathing.

Asthma. Palpitation of the heart, with a feeling of suffocation.

Dropsy of the chest.

Ulcers, with *burning* pain.

Scaly eruptions, as dry salt rheum, Blue spots. Black blisters, burning and painful. Putrid ulcers, with fetid discharge. Proud flesh.

ATROPINE.

Much the same as *Bell.*, but more efficacious

in many nervous affections, especially nervous headache, coming on suddenly.

BELLADONNA.

Spasms of the limbs, with delirium. Convulsions Excessive sensibility of the organs of sense.

Swelling of the glands. Ulcers, burning when touched.

Erysipelas, especially of the head and face.

Chilblains, red and burning.

Drowsiness and stupor. Deep, lethargic sleep, with snoring.

During fever, delirum; red face and violent thirst.

All sorts of delirium and craziness, singing, talking, laughing, crying, quarreling, raging, biting.

Dizziness and intoxicated feeling.

Headache, as if the brain was stunned. Feeling of great weight and heaviness of the brain. Pressive headache in the forehead, preventing opening of the eyes, increased by motion. Throbbing headache. Feeling of swashing in the brain.

Heat and redness of the face, with violent headache; when stooping the blood rushes to the head.

Face bluish red, or dark red.

Inflammation of the eyes. One sees objects double or wrong side up. Dilated pupils.

Tongue red, hot, dry, cracked.

Inflammation of the throat and glands.

Contractive griping in the abdomen. Long, lasting pain in the whole abdomen, as if sore and raw.

Urgent bearing down in women, followed by discharge of mucous leucorrhœa. Leucorrhœa with colic. Inflammation and painful swelling of the breasts. Erysipelas of the breasts.

Hoarseness, noise and rattling in the bronchial tubes. Every breath causes dry cough. Night cough. Violent dry cough. Whooping cough.

BRYONIA.

Every part of the body on which one is lying, aches.

Sleeplessness from heat, but when one uncovers he feels cold.

Delirium at night. Somnambulism. Nightmare.

Chilliness and shuddering, followed by dry heat, then sweat. Sour sweat.

Headache, which does not begin when waking, but when opening and moving the eyes.

The blood rushes to the head, and the head feels compressed from temple to temple. Violent headache; the head feels very heavy. Headache when stooping, as if all the contents of the head would issue through the forehead. The headache begins chiefly in the morning; is aggravated by motion, especially by opening and moving the eyes.

The scalp is sore and painful to the touch.

Dryness of the mouth; tongue coated white or yellow.

Dry, sore throat, with hoarseness. Sticking sensation in the throat when swallowing, turning the head or touching the throat.

Pain, and sensation of swelling in the region of the stomach.

Tightness, burning or stinging, in the region of the liver, when touching it, when coughing or taking a long breath.

Soreness and bloating of the abdomen.

Dropsy of the abdomen. Constipation.

Hot urine, red or brown, and scanty.

Hoarseness and roughness of voice when in the open air. Hoarseness with easy sweating.

Dry cough. Vomiting of food when coughing. Sensation when coughing as if the head and chest would fly to pieces.

Burning pain in the right half of the chest. The breathing is short and hurried. Cough, difficult breathing and mucous or bloody expectoration. Inflammation of the lungs. Pleurisy.

Rheumatism. A great variety of rheumatic pains in the back and limbs, with or without redness and swelling.

CALCAREA.

Is best adapted to children of a plethoric, scrofulous or rickety constitution, who have a tendency to cold in the head, sore eyes or diarrhœa; tedious and difficult teething; weak limbs and slowness in learning to walk. Also, to plethoric or feeble women, who menstruate too frequently and too profusely.

Great weakness and sensitiveness to cold air, and great liability to take cold.

Unhealthy skin, so that small wounds or scratches inflame and ulcerate and do not heal.

Chaps and cracks in the hands and lips.

Palpitation of the heart, with weakness.

Exhausting sweat, day and night, Sweat from the slightest exercise. Night sweats. Internal chilliness.

Melancholy, low spirited, and apprehensive. Great inclination to weep. Changeable mood. The head is easily affected by mental labor.

Headache every morning on waking. Pain of one side of the head. Pain and pressure in the top of the head. Pain in the back of the head, as if pressed assunder. Throbbing pain in the middle of the brain every morning. Inflammation, redness and ulceration of the nose. Dryness, stoppage and bad smell from the nose.

Thin pale face, with dark-bordered eyes.

Swelling of the upper lip in the morning.

Swelling and bleeding of the gums. Blisters in the mouth and on the tongue.

Weakness and sleepiness after dinner or supper. Violent beating of the heart after dinner. Pain and fullness in the abdomen and liver.

Constant gurgling in the abdomen.

Obstinate constipation in feeble constitutions.

Diarrhœa in scrofulous or consumptive persons.

Too frequent and *profuse* menstruation. During menstruation, rush of blood to the head; heat in the head and painful pressure in the top of the head; or toothache. After menstruation, milk-like or burning and itching leucorrhœa.

Bearing down in the lower part of the back.

Sweat of the knees and of the feet. Burning or pain and soreness in the soles of the feet.

CALENDULA.

This is an essential remedy as an external application in wounds, when the flesh or skin is broken or cut. It prevents inflammation, and greatly hastens the healing. Also in old suppurating, inflamed, and painful ulcers and sores.

CAMPHOR.

Coldness and chilliness. Cold sweat. Small, weak pulse. Pale face. Spasms of the muscles of the mouth, and frothing. Dim vision.

Cholera, with cramps, coldness, anguish and burning, and pains at the pit of the stomach.

Pain and difficulty in urinating.

Slow, panting breathing; oppression of the chest, and feeling of suffocation. Spasms of the chest.

Fainting.

CANNABIS SAT.

Opacity of the cornea. Specks on the cornea.

Piercing headache. Headache in the top of the head, as if a stone were pressing on it.

Painful pressure in the forehead, temple and eyelids.

Pain in the region of the kidneys. Pain and difficulty in urinating. Burning pain along the passage when urinating. Bloody urine. Discharges of mucus.

CANTHARIS.

Erysipelas, with burning and blisters. Heat and burning in the stomach and abdomen. Pains in the kidneys, and along the passage from the kidneys to the bladder. Extreme pain, burning and difficulty in urinating. Violent pain, heat and burning in the bladder, and difficult and painful urination. Constant and urgent desire to urinate, passing a few drops with great pain. Urine bloody. Entire suppression of urine. The urine passes involuntarily. Wetting the bed, in children.

CARBO VEG.

Is adapted to the following symptoms in persons weak and debilitated. Rheumatic, drawing pains in the limbs and whole body and great weakness after the pains. The limbs go to sleep, feel bruised, and the joints are weak.

Burning of the skin in different parts. Nettle rash. Great disposition to sweat. Morning and night sweats, with weakness.

Peevish, irritable and whining mood.

Aching on top and back of the head, with pain when the hair is touched. Beating headache. Buzzing in the ear. Falling out of the hair, after sickness.

Black, flying spots before the eyes.

The complexion becomes very yellow or very pale. After eating or drinking, fullness of the abdomen, and headache.

Diarrhœa, with burning, smarting and aching in the rectum. Wind colic.

Burning in the soles, or profuse sweat of the feet.

CAULOPHYLLUM.

Nervous sleeplessness in weak females. Rheumatic headache.

Nursing sore mouth.

Full, pressed feeling of the uterus. Drawing in the groins. Labor-like pains. Premature pains, threatening miscarriage. False, wrangling pains. After-pains.

Painful menstruation.

Taken for some weeks before confinement, it renders labor more easy.

Rheumatism of the small joints, feet, hands, legs and arms.

CHAMOMILLA.

Convulsions of children. Weeping, moaning and starting in sleep.

Great thirst, and dry, red tongue.

Chilliness in the open air, or when uncovered.

Night or morning sweat, without sleep.

Tendency to weep, and start. Crying on account of a very trifling, and often imaginary offense. Peevish; is unable to stop talking about old vexations.

Excessive sensitiveness to odors.

Headache as if it would burst, on walking. The head feels bruised.

Toothache, aggravated by anything warm in the mouth, or a warm room.

Sour, bitter or putrid taste of the mouth.

Sour eructations, fullness after a meal, and then nausea and vomiting.

Wind colic; fullness of the abdomen, which feels bruised. Colic, with light-colored stools. Hot diarrhœic stools, smelling like rotten eggs. Discharges of white or green mucus, with colic.

Yellow, corrosive leucorrhœa, or acrid and watery. Pressing down, like labor pains.

Before menstruation, cutting colic; abdominal spasms and drawing in the thighs.

Cramps in the calves.

CHINA.

Weakness and other affections, attending the loss of blood, and other fluids.

Excessive sensibility of the nervous system, with great weakness.

Languor and exhausted state of body and mind. Easy sweating.

Headache, pressive, tearing or throbbing, increased by stepping, or a current of air. Pain and soreness of the scalp. Sweat of the head. Face pale, sickly and sunken. Lips dry, parched and chapped, or blackish.

Yellow skin. Jaundice.

Drowsiness in the day, and restless sleep at night.

Tongue coated white, yellow or dirty. Loss of appetite. Taste flat, insipid or bitter. Desire for various things, without knowing what. Desire for wine or sour things.

Hungry, with nausea. Fullness after eating.

Pain in the region of the liver, when touched. Swelling of the liver, and spleen.

Undigested, blackish, bilious or white stools.

Excessive menstruation of weakly women, with discharges of clots of black blood.

CINA.

Bronchial catarrh and cough, remaining after measles.

Convulsions, and contortions of the limbs.

Epileptic convulsions, without loss of consciousness. The child tosses from side to side; restless, whether asleep or awake.

Weeping and complaining.

Disposition to bore in the nose, and rub the nose. Stoppage of the nose.

Pale face, and sickly appearance around the eyes. Grinding the teeth.

Changeable appetite—sometimes voracious.

Vomiting and diarrhœa after drinking.

Cutting pain in the abdomen. Vomiting of worms. Diarrhœa, and itching of the anus.

Various complaints, arising from worms.

N. B.—*Cina* takes the place of *Santonine* in former editions of this work.

Copious, frequent urination. Turbid urine. Wetting the bed in children.

Tickling low down in the throat, producing cough. Before coughing, the child raises itself suddenly; the whole body looks rigid; it is without consciousness, as if it would have an epileptic fit. The child moans after coughing.

Violent hunger, shortly after a meal.

COCCULUS.

Absorbed in reveries and sad thoughts. Restless eagerness to do something.

Headache, with nausea.

Nausea from riding in a carriage, with colic.

Painful menstruation, with discharge of coagulated blood.

COFFEA.

Great nervousness. Sleeplessness, owing to agitation of body and mind.

Frequent yawning.

Sensitiveness to cold, and aversion to open air.

Pain on one side of the head, as if a nail had been driven into the skull.

Headache, as if the brain were torn, and would be dashed to pieces, coming on during a walk in the open air, and subsiding in a room. Pain in the head, as if too full.

Diarrhœa during teething.

Crampy sensation in the calves and feet.

COLOCYNTH.

Spasmodic pain of the stomach, extending into the throat, with nausea. Sharp griping in the abdomen. Griping about the umbilicus, like cutting or squeezing; worse on moving, and relieved on bending forward. Feeling as if the intestines were squeezed between stones, and would burst.

Wind colic. Bilious colic.

Diarrhœa, and straining at stool. Dysentery. Frequent stools, with nausea.

Mucous stools, or liquid and frothy, of yellow color and musty odor.

Itching, burning, soreness and rawness of the anus, after stool.

CROTON.

Scarlet redness of the skin, with rashlike vesicles. Itching, followed by painful burning. Itch.

Burning inflammation of the mouth, lips and throat as if burnt.

Great flatulence of the bowels.

Fullness, pressure and burning in the stomach and bowels. Piercing and cutting in the bowels.

Numerous liquid stools, with straining. Violent purging.

The urine looks dark and fiery, with greasy particles floating on the top, and producing burning in passing.

CUPRUM MET.

Cramps and convulsions. Deep sleep with jerking of the limbs.

Convulsive laughter. Craziness, with merry singing. Artful craziness.

Vomiting. Violent vomiting with diarrhœa.

Vomiting, with colic. Cholera, with cramps.

Spasms in the abdomen, with colic.

Violent diarrhœa. Spasms in the throat. Cough like whooping cough, arresting the breathing. Spasmodic asthma.

DROSERA.

Tickling in the throat, with short, hacking cough. Rough, scraping feeling of dryness in the throat, with cough and hoarseness. Pain below the ribs when coughing. Cough so rapid and hurried that he is out of breath. Whooping cough; the cough causes vomiting and nose bleed.

DULCAMARA.

Eruption of the skin, like nettlerash. Eruption forming crusts over the body.

Slimy diarrhœa, from a cold.

Urine thick and white, or reddish and burning. Red or white sediment in the urine.

Difficult and painful urination. Catarrh of the bladder, and discharge of mucus, with the urine. Cough, with expectoration of tough mucus, with stiches in the chest.

GELSEMIUM.

Irritability. Dull, stupid, intoxicated feeling of the head.

Dull, stupefying, pressive headache. Dizziness.

Heaviness of the eyelids; difficult keeping the eyes open; dim, blurred vision. Double vision. Dilated pupils.

Cold in the head, with sneezing and watery discharges from the nose. Influenza. Measles.

Chilliness, as in the begining of colds, fevers, and many inflammatory affections.

Chills, with headache and pains in the back and limbs.

Scarlet fever. Bilious fever, (early stage.)

Excessive and tedious labor pains. After-pains.

GRAPHITES,

Spots on the skin like flea bites. Small, red, itching pimples. Small boils on the neck, back and arms.

Unhealthy skin; small injuries inflame and suppurate.

Night sweat; fetid and sour sweat.

Itching of the hairy scalp. Scabs on the head. Moist eruptions on the top of the head, painful to the touch. Scrufy spots on the head. Falling of the hair.

Single hairs get gray.

Bad smelling discharge from the ears.

Sore feeling in the nose, when blowing it. Black, sweaty pores on the nose. Dry scurfs in the nose. Sore, cracked ulcerated, nostrils. Bad smell from the nose. Obstruction of the nose.

Erysipelas of the face; freckles.

Ulcerated corners of the mouth.

Eruption on the chin.

Profuse leucorrhœa, mucous or thin.

The toe and finger nails are thick, rough and deformed.

HAMAMELIS.

Bleeding from the nose, stomach, bowels, lungs, uterus and bladder; the blood being usually dark. Bloody dysentery. Piles. Milk leg. Inflammation and enlargement of the veins of the legs and other parts.

HEPAR SULPHUR.

Fine stinging, burning, itching. Nettle rash. Chapped skin of the hands and feet. Slight injuries become sore and suppurate. Ulcers bleed easily.

Redness and swelling of the upper eyelid. Styes. Running of fetid pus from the ears.

Eruptions about the mouth. Itching pimples on the chin.

Looseness of the teeth—the gums bleed easily.

Smarting roughness and rawness of the throat. Stinging and stitches in the throat—sometimes extending to the ears.

Fetid sweats in the arm pits.

Cough, from scraping and roughness of the throat.

Perhaps the best remedy for felon; chilblains.

HYDRASTIS.

Old ulcers. Small pox. Running from the ears. Cancer.

Swelling of the eyelids, with discharge of pus,

and sticking together of the eyelids. (*External and internal use.*)

Obstinate catarrh, (*used internally and snuffed.*)

Canker of the mouth. Nursing sore mouth.

Ulcerated throat, (*as a gargle.*) Diphtheria.

Dyspepsia, with weakness of the stomach.

Chronic, mucous diarrhœa. Obstinate constipation.

IGNATIA.

Jerks in the limbs when going to sleep. Restless sleep, with night-mare. Moaning in sleep. Snoring. Excessive convulsive yawning.

Anxious desire to do things in haste; hurriedness.

Impatient — intolerant of contradiction, or noise.

Still, serious melancholy. Brooding to himself.

Great grief at loss of friends.

Ulcerated nostrils, or pain as if ulcerated.

The lips crack and bleed. Ulceration in the corners of the mouth.

Stinging in the throat when not swallowing. Sensation when swallowing as if one swallowed over a lump. Stinging sore throat.

Rough, dry cough, especially after measles.

IPECAC.

Rigid stretching of the body in children. Chilliness, but unable to bear warmth.

Peevish, impatient; unable to bear the least noise.

Headache, as if the brain and skull were

bruised, through all the bones, down to the root of the tongue, with nausea.

Yellowish or white coating of the tongue.

Sweet taste, as of blood in the mouth.

Bitter taste. Nausea and vomiting.

Vomiting of food or mucus; yellow, green or jelly-like or of black, pitch-like substance. Sense of great emptiness and goneness of the stomach.

Wind colic, with diarrhœa.

Stool green as grass, or fermented, like yeast.

Fetid stools. Stools covered with bloody mucus.

Liquid diarrhœa, with nausea. Bloody stools.

Bloody urine. Turbid urine, with brick-dust sediment.

Uterine hemorrhage.

Rattling of mucus in the bronchial tubes.

Suffocative cough. Cough from tickling in the throat and through the chest.

Bleeding from the lungs.

Spasmodic asthma.

KALI BICHROMICUM.

Excessive weakness, and small pulse. Soreness of the nose, with watery discharge, and sneezing. Stoppage and ulceration of the nose.

Loss of smell.

Tongue smooth, red and cracked.

Scraping of the throat. Throat sore, red, swollen, painful and finally ulcerated.

Important in diphtheria, ulcerated throat and membranous croup.

Tickling in the throat, causing cough.

Loud wheezing cough, with retching and expectoration of tough mucus. Chronic loud cough. Loud wheezing and rattling in the chest.

Difficult breathing, with expectoration of white mucus as tough as pitch.

KALI HYDRIODICUM.

Profuse, dry eruption on the face, on the shoulders and over the whole body.

Catarrhal fever.

Burning in the eyes, with secretion of yellow mucus. Burning and redness of the lids, and itching.

Redness and swelling of nose. Discharge of burning, acrid water from the nose.

Profuse watery discharge from the nose.

Dry, chapped lips. Ulceration of the tongue and mouth.

Sore throat. Dull, stinging pains in the throat.

Thin, watery, acrid leucorrhœa.

Hoarseness, cough, soreness of the bronchia and oppressed breathing.

Influenza, with sneezing, headache and drowsiness.

Irritation of the throat, with dry cough, followed by copious, greenish expectoration.

LEPTANDRIN.

Bilious headache, with coated tongue, bitter taste, and low spirits.

Dull aching in the region of the liver, extending to the back. Jaundice, with light clay-colored stools. Stool followed by a feeling of weakness of the bowels and rectum. Stools hard, black and lumpy, then soft and mushy.

Great rumbling and distress in the lower bowels, with profuse, black, fetid stools.

Mucous, bloody stools.

MACROTIN.

Nervous, rheumatic and menstrual headache. Dull pain in the back of the head and neck. Leucorrhœa. Excessive menstruation. Suppressed menses. Weight and bearing down of the uterine region and back.

Labor-like pains during pregnancy. Spinal irritation.

Rheumatism in the back and limbs.

MERCURIUS.

Inflammation of the eyes, with itching, burning, swelling and redness. Scurf round the eyes. Running of water and pus from the eyes, and sticking together of the lids. Ulcer on the cornea.

Pain and discharge from the ears.

Swelling of the nose. Sneezing and running of the nose.

Ulcerations and cracks in the corners of the mouth.

Swelling and ulcerations of the gums. Sore

mouth; cancer; salivation. Swelling of the tongue.

Sore throat. Pain when swallowing. Ulcers in the throat. Diphtheria.

Inflammation and pain in the liver. Jaundice.

Colic and diarrhœa, pain worse by walking. and chilliness. Inflammation of the bowels.

Diarrhœa, with chilliness, and urging at stool.

Dysentery.

Brown urine; dark red as if mixed with blood.

Constant desire to urinate.

Catarrh, with chilliness, sore throat and running at the nose.

Swelling of the glands of the neck, arm pits and groins.

N. B.—*Merc. cor.* is usually preferable in dysentery. In other cases *Merc. sol.* is preferred for women and children, and *Merc. cor.* for men.

Merc. iodatus is preferable to either in diphtheria, and some forms of ulcerated throat.

NUX VOMICA.

Chronic ailments from the use of wine, spirituous liquors, coffee and other narcotics, and from watching.

Pain in all the joints, as if bruised; worse from motion. Paralysis and trembling of the limbs. Trembling of drunkards. Convulsions and spasms. Bending the head and body backwards. St. Vitus dance.

Chilblains, itching, and burning.

Great chilliness; sometimes with hot head and face, and headache.

Burning, internal heat and thirst.

Starting on going to sleep. Horrid dreams.

Sour night sweat. Morning sweat.

Great sensitiveness to all external impressions.

Noise, talk, strong odors and bright light are intolerable.

Headache, from stormy weather, wine or coffee; from thinking; piles from sedentary habits. Headache, with nausea. Headache on one side.

Stoppage of the nose.

Earthy, yellowish complexion.

Cankered mouth. Sour taste. Milk sours.

Putrid taste. Hungry, but aversion to food.

After a meal, sick feeling, as if he had overloaded his stomach; low spirits; chilly; hot face; dull headache; sleepiness and nausea.

Hiccough; bitter or sour eructation; heartburn,

Pressure in the stomach, as from a stone.

Fullness and throbbing in the liver. Jaundice.

Constipation from sedentary habits.

Mucous diarrhœa. After stools, burning and smarting in the rectum. Piles, burning and pricking.

Painful discharge of thick urine; burning and pricking.

Internal swelling of the vagina, like prolapsus.

The menses appear too early. During the menses, nausea, chilliness, fainting and headache.

Yellow leucorrhœa.

Nausea and vomiting during pregnancy.

Symptoms of miscarriage. False labor pains.

Colds, with headache; heat in the face; Chilliness and scraping in the throat and chest, with hawking.

Dry, fatiguing, continuous cough.

Bruised pain in the back. Stiffness of the back and neck.

PHOSPHORUS.

Hectic fever, night sweats.

Pale, sickly, or sunken, livid countenance.

Sore throat, with dark redness, burning and dry.

Burning in the stomach.

Chronic diarrhœa; also of consumptive persons.

Alternate constipation and diarrhœa of old persons.

Burning, gnawing and itching in the rectum.

Colds, with roughness of the throat and windpipe.

Violent cold, with hoarseness, cough and fever.

Expectoration of tough or reddish mucus.

Inflammation of the lungs.

PHOSPHORIC ACID.

Pains in the bones and weakness of the young who are growing rapidly.

Profuse morning sweat.

Scurf on the nose and large pimples on the face.

Diarrhœa, with rumbling and pain. Watery diarrhœa, or white-gray. Passage of undigested food.

Milky urine.

PHODOPHYLLIN.

Pains in the bowels, followed by diarrhœa.

Fullness, pain and soreness in the region of the liver.

Diarrhœa in the morning, or after eating.

Diarrhœa, with screaming, in children, when teething.

Green, white, slimy or hot, watery stools, with great weakness. Undigested stools. Dark-yellow mucous stools, smelling like carrion. Chalk-like stools, with gagging and thirst in children.

Chronic diarrhœa, worse in the morning.

Falling of the bowel in children. Piles.

Leucorrhœa, thick, transparent. Prolapsus uteri.

PULSATILLA.

Restless sleep, with dry, burning heat. Disposed to weep or cough. Gloomy; peevish; sullen; chilly.

Headache deep in the orbits, when moving the eyes,

Headache, as if from intoxication, or watching or as from overloading the stomach, or from fat meat.

Redness and swelling of the edges of the eyelids. Stye.

Earache. Hardness of hearing. Discharge from the ears.

Green, fetid discharge from the nose.

Toothache when taking anything warm in the mouth.

Slimy taste, or taste of putrid meat.

The middle of the tongue feels as if burnt.

Nausea. Vomiting, sour, salt or bitter.

Food tastes bitter. Waterbrash. Eructations, tasting of the food, or sour, bitter or bilious.

Urging to stool, as if diarrhœa would set in.

Suppressed menses, with nausea and vomiting.

Before the menses, chilliness, stretching, yawning and heaviness of the abdomen.

During the menses, pain of the stomach; pressure in the abdomen and back; chilliness and pale face.

The blood is thick, black and clotty.

Leucorrhœa; burning, or thin and acrid; or milky, or thick and mucous. Swelling of the breast, and excessive secretion of milk, when weaning.

Cough, with difficult expectoration of yellow mucus, or bitter. Cough, with putrid expectoration and hectic fever.

RHUS TOX.

Rheumatism, with stiffness and weakness of the joints, with stinging pains.

Swelling or redness on or near the joints.

Rheumatism of the hip joint and wrist.

The greatest stiffness and pain are felt on first moving the joints after rest, and in the morning.

Bad effects from straining parts. Pains as if sprained.

Greatest sensitiveness to the open air.

Burning, itching eruptions of vesicles.

Nettle rash. Shingles. Erysipelas, with blisters. Swelling of glands.

Evening fever, with diarrhœa.

Inflammation of the eyelids. Gluing of the eyes together. Red, hard stye on the lids.

Milk crusts.

Parched, red, dry tongue.

Diarrhœa. Red and yellow stools, mixed with mucus, jelly-like, and fluid. Stools mixed with blood.

SEPIA.

Is an important remedy for females. Ringworm. Flushes of heat.

Palpitation of the heart, in the evening in bed and beating of all the arteries.

Profuse night sweat. Cold night sweat on the chest back and thighs. Sourish night sweat. Morning sweat. Sweat from the least exertion.

Despondent; sad; indifferent. Sensitive to noise.

Dizziness only when walking.

Morning headache, with nausea. Beating

headache in the evening. Headache as if the head would burst, and the eyes fall out.

Pain in the scalp, when touching it.

Great falling off of the hair.

Small red pimples on the forehead. Rough forehead.

Yellow spots on the face. Black pores on the face. Yellowness round the mouth.

Pain of the tongue, as if burnt and blistered.

Everything tastes too salt.

Heat and palpitation of the heart, after eating. Morning nausea.

Vomiting, during pregnancy.

Exhausting diarrhœa; green or sour in children, or putrid, sourish, fetid smell.

Slimy diarrhœa, with distended abdomen.

Itching and stinging in the rectum.

Prolapsus of the uterus and vagina.

Before the menses, colic and faintness, shuddering, and acrid leucerrhœa, producing soreness.

During the menses, exhustion, toothache, pain in the limbs, spasms in the abdomen and pressing downward.

Leucorrhœa, with stiches in the uterus, or with itching in the vagina. Bloody mucus; yellowish, watery or mucous leucorrhœa.

Discharge of a greenish, red fluid, during pregnancy.

Leucorrhœa like milk, only in the day time, producing soreness.

During pregnancy—toothache, nausea and vomiting, and stinging in the breast.

Sprained weary feeling in the small of the back.

Violent cramps in the calves at night.

Profuse sweat of the feet. Burning of the feet at night. Fetid smell of the feet.

SPONGIA.

Stinging in the throat. Hoarseness, cough and running at the nose. Scraping and burning at the throat. Difficult breathing, as if the throat were closed by a plug. Hollow cough, day and night. Pain in the chest and windpipe, when coughing, with roughness in the throat. Constant cough, from a deep spot in the chest where a pain is felt, as if sore. Croup.

SULPHUR.

Scurfy eruptions, itching.

Stinging, itching rash. Milk crusts.

Nettle rash, with fever. Burning, itching eruptions.

Liver spots on the chest and back; itching.

Yellow brown spots. Dry, scaly eruptions.

Unhealthy skin. Boils.

Swelling, suppuration, or hardness of glands.

Disease of bones.

Low spirits. Extremely forgetful.

Pain in the center of the head, from coughing or sneezing. Pain in the top of the head as if the eyes would be pressed down.

Scald head, or fetid and moist eruption with thick pus, yellow crust, and itching.

Itching of the eyelids. Painful dryness of the eyeballs. Heat or bruised pain in the eyes.

Running of matter from the eyes.

Ulceration of the nose. Dryness. Loss of smell.

Chapped lips. Eruption around the mouth.

Chronic constipation, and with piles; lumpy stools, mixed with mucus, with burning pain in the rectum. Scalding, hot stools.

Burning in the vagina, and itching in the external parts.

Burning, painful leucorrhœa, producing soreness.

Dry cough, only when in the open air.

Dry night cough. Coughing up greenish lumps.

TARTAR EMETIC.

Violent itching and suppurating rash.

Round, large, burning, painful pustules, surrounded by a red circle. Boil-like pustules, with violent, painful itching. Pustules containing a bloody or blackish fluid. Small pox.

Fever with restlessness; chilliness, alternating with heat; great heat and thirst; Muttering delirum. Headache and palpitation of the heart; Dullness; drowsy and weary feeling.

The eyeballs feel bruised and sore. Influenza. Dryness of the lips and mouth. Red tongue, covered with raised, red points.

Sore throat, with burning heat of throat.

Loathing of food; nausea. Vomiting and diarrhœa.

Feeble voice. Cough and sneezing.

Short and difficult breathing. Inflammation

of the lungs, with continued dry, or loose, rattling cough; cannot breath lying down.

Velvety feeling of the chest.

VERATRUM ALBUM.

Blue skin in cholera. Coldness of the body. Cold sweat. Sweat, with burning skin.

Headache, with nausea, vomiting and pale face.

Chilly on the top of the head.

Cold sweat on the forehead.

Cold disfigured face, as of a dead person.

Redness of face when lying down and pale when sitting up.

Tongue dry, blackish and cracked.

Desire for fruit and acid things. Intense thirst.

Nausea before breakfast. Nausea, with bitter taste.

Hiccough. Drinking is followed by shuddering or goose skin.

Great nausea, with thirst. Vomiting of bile, of food and of mucus, with great weakness.

Black vomit. Cholera. Cholera morbus. Coldness or burning of the stomach.

Voilent diarrhœa, with chilliness. Extreme weakness during the stools.

Scanty, burning, yellow, turbid or dark-red urine.

Cramps of the calves. Icy cold feet.

INDEX.

www.ingramcontent.com/pod-product-compliance
Lightning Source LLC
LaVergne TN
LVHW021414110826
845150LV00007B/1915